Adrian Vega

Arcturian Holistic Healing System
Guide to Multidimensional Healing
and the Awakening of Consciousness

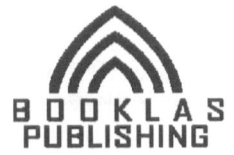

Original title: Sistema Holístico de Sanación Arcturiana

Copyright © 2025, published by Luiz Antonio dos Santos ME.

This book presents the fundamental principles of Reiki, exploring its historical roots, energy practices, and impact on physical, emotional, and spiritual well-being. Through accessible language and practical examples, the work guides readers on a journey of self-discovery and inner healing.

1st Edition

Production Team
Author: Adrian Vega
Editor: Luiz Santos
Review: Anacleto Borba
Cover: Studios Booklas / Tadeu Sheller
Translation: Anselmo Costa Neto

Publication and Identification
Arcturian Holistic Healing System / By Adrian Vega
Booklas Publishing, 2024
Categories: Body, Mind and Spirit / Health and Healing / Meditation
DDC: 615.852 - CDU: 613.8
ISBN: 978-65-9981-024-4

All rights reserved to:
Booklas Publishing / Luiz Antonio dos Santos ME
No part of this book may be reproduced, stored in a retrieval system, or transmitted by any means - electronic, mechanical, photocopying, recording, or otherwise - without the prior and express permission of the copyright holder.

Summary

Prologue 5
Chapter 1 Arcturian Multidimensional Healing 7
Chapter 2 Energy and Vibrational Anatomy 14
Chapter 3 Preparation and Holistic Healing 22
Chapter 4 Frequencies and Creative Power 32
Chapter 5 Connection and Sacred Tools 41
Chapter 6 Connection and Sacred Tools 50
Chapter 7 Ethics and Energy Purification 58
Chapter 8 Chakras and Self-Healing 66
Chapter 9 Sacred Geometry and Channeling 74
Chapter 10 Auric Healing and Protection 82
Chapter 11 Mental and Energy Healing 90
Chapter 12 Remote Healing and Sacred Spaces 99
Chapter 13 Multidimensional Healing and Energy Fusion 107
Chapter 14 Collective Healing and Intuition 115
Chapter 15 Crystals and Arcturian Healing 123
Chapter 16 Activation of the Light Body 131
Chapter 17 Reprogramming and Interdimensional Healing 139
Chapter 18 Arcturian Masters and Symbols 147
Chapter 19 Reconstruction of Energetic DNA and Ancestral Healing 155
Chapter 20 Sound and Heart Healing 163
Chapter 21 Cosmic Alignment and Animal Healing 171
Chapter 22 Energy Protection and Release 179
Chapter 23 Healing Relationships and Light 186

Chapter 24 Harmony with the Earth and Regeneration 194
Chapter 25 Child and Group Healing 201
Chapter 26 Mastery and Advanced Practice 209
Epilogue 216

Prologue

From the depths of the cosmos, where silence is interrupted only by the vibrational melody of the universe, an undeniable invitation arises: a journey into your interior, beyond the barriers imposed by the mind and body. What you are about to hold is not just a book; it is a map, a guide, and a key. Each page has been imbued with a singular purpose: to awaken within you the resonance of something that has always been there, waiting for the right moment to emerge.

The Arcturians, beings of wisdom and light, have opened a window through this knowledge, connecting to what is most subtle and pure in you. Their frequencies and energies, which transcend conventional understanding, resonate with what we call essence, the point of balance between the physical and the spiritual. They do not present themselves as distant masters, but as companions who recognize the infinite potential of your existence.

Throughout your life, you may have felt an inexplicable emptiness, a constant search for something you never found. You may have noticed that the answers you sought were always one step beyond where you looked. This book, however, is different. It was written for you—not for the collective, not for a crowd, but for your unique soul, with its challenges, dreams, and potentialities.

Arcturian holistic medicine is not just a remedy for the body. It is a reminder that everything within you is connected: mind, spirit, emotions, and physical body. You carry within you an energy system that pulsates with the truths of the universe. Each block you release, each wound you heal, generates a new melody that aligns with the purest frequency of the cosmos.

In the following pages, you will not only find information, but also vibrations that activate dormant parts of your consciousness. Each practice, each concept, each teaching has been designed to make you remember, to ignite within you the power you have always had, but which may have been silenced by the density of the world.

Allow this reading to be more than an intellectual act. Feel it. Connect with it. For in doing so, not only will your energy system align, but the universe around you will also change. That is the power you carry within you. And this book is a reminder that you are never alone on this path.

Luiz Santos
Editor

Chapter 1
Arcturian Multidimensional Healing

Holistic healing isn't simply a healing process; it's a transformative experience that encompasses every corner of our existence. In the vast fabric of life, everything is interconnected: body, mind, emotions, and spirit form a delicate balance that sustains our well-being. This multidimensional healing system transcends conventional barriers to offer us a path to true inner harmony.

At the heart of this approach is the understanding that each aspect of our existence reflects a greater whole. Physical illnesses are often an echo of emotional imbalances, while energy blocks can manifest as intrusive thoughts or even diseases. Recognizing this intricate interrelationship is the first step towards authentic healing, which not only alleviates symptoms but heals the root of our ailments.

Arcturian healing emerges as a holistic system that integrates these dimensions, guiding us to a state of deep balance. It is essential to understand the foundations upon which it is based. The term "holistic healing" evokes the image of an integrated whole, but what does it actually mean? In essence, it is about approaching the human being as an indivisible whole. While conventional medical practices tend to focus on isolated symptoms, the holistic approach explores the underlying causes at all levels: physical, emotional, mental, and spiritual. This paradigm seeks not only to alleviate suffering but to restore the vitality inherent in each individual.

On this journey, the Arcturians play a unique role. These high vibrational beings, known for their deep spiritual and energetic knowledge, offer us tools and teachings that resonate with the highest frequencies of the cosmos. Their connection to humanity is not accidental, but a relationship cultivated over millennia, designed to guide us to a greater understanding of our place in the universe and our innate capacity to heal.

Arcturian healing is, in essence, a journey of self-discovery. Before we learn to channel these energies, we must examine our own internal energies. What thought patterns dominate our mind? What emotions do we repress? What signals does our body send us that we ignore? Each of these aspects offers crucial clues to understanding the state of our being and the path to healing.

The multidimensionality of this system lies in its ability to address these issues from multiple perspectives. Imagine that your being is like a musical instrument, with each aspect of your existence representing a string. When these strings are tuned and vibrate in unison, the music they produce is harmonious and balanced. But if one string is out of tune, the whole melody is affected. Holistic healing acts as the tuner that restores lost harmony.

In this process, we seek not only to heal the body, but also to release trapped emotions, reprogram harmful mental patterns, and reconnect with our spiritual essence. It is a dance between the visible and invisible dimensions of our existence, in which each step brings us closer to our natural state of well-being.

Holistic healing also invites us to recognize our interconnection with the environment around us. We live in a vibrational universe, where every thought, emotion, and action generates waves that affect the fabric of reality. Just as a river flows harmoniously when it is free of obstacles, our vital energy flows better when we are in balance. But when this flow is interrupted, whether by stress, trauma, or external influences, blockages arise that impact our health.

This is where the Arcturian teachings offer their wisdom. Connected to the purest frequencies of the universe, these practices teach us to release blockages and restore the natural flow of energy. It is not a simple act of healing, but a return to our original state of balance.

As we delve deeper into this path, we begin to understand that healing is not an isolated event, but a continuous process of transformation. Each experience, each challenge, and each triumph are opportunities to grow and realign ourselves with our highest essence.

Arcturian healing not only empowers us to heal, but also to become agents of transformation, radiating balance and harmony to everything around us. From this starting point, the reader is invited to explore the depths of their being, to connect with universal energies, and to discover the immense healing potential that resides within each of us. Holistic healing is not a destination, but a continuous journey to wholeness, and the path begins here.

In the vast expanses of the cosmos, where stars shine like beacons of eternity, there are civilizations that have transcended physical limitations and achieved a state of pure vibration. The Arcturians are one such elevated collective, known for their deep commitment to spiritual expansion and energetic balance in the universe. Their name comes from the star Arcturus, located in the constellation Bootes, a beacon of light that resonates with a frequency of love, wisdom, and healing.

Unlike entities that inhabit the dense planes of existence, Arcturians are not limited by physical bodies in the sense that we understand them. Instead, they operate on higher levels of consciousness, where matter and energy coexist in perfect harmony. Although they can assume forms perceived by humans in meditative experiences or channeling, their true nature is vibrational, composed of frequencies that resonate with the highest levels of creation.

Their connection to humanity is not a recent phenomenon, but a bond cultivated over eons. Since ancient times, the Arcturians have guided human civilizations, acting as guardians of knowledge and healing. Through messages transmitted in dreams, deep meditation, or altered states of consciousness, they have imparted wisdom about the workings of the universe, the power of energy, and the path to spiritual evolution.

Often, these connections manifest as a gentle inner calling, a sense of inexplicable familiarity, or visions of geometric shapes and luminous patterns. Those who have responded to this call describe a feeling of deep peace, as if returning to a spiritual home they had forgotten. The Arcturians, with their infinite patience, are always present for those who seek to understand their purpose and achieve higher levels of balance.

The mission of the Arcturians transcends the human plane. As universal guardians, they are deeply committed to preserving energy balance throughout the cosmos. This commitment includes assisting civilizations in transition, especially those facing periods of crisis or significant evolution. In the case of Earth, their goal is to help humanity awaken to its true potential, reminding us that we are multidimensional beings capable of co-creating our reality.

In the context of healing, the Arcturians act as catalysts for transformation. Their energy operates on subtle levels, penetrating the deepest energy blockages and promoting a vibrational alignment that restores the natural flow of vital energy. It is not a direct intervention, but a cooperation between their high frequencies and the conscious intention of the receiver. In this way, they empower us to be active participants in our healing process.

The Arcturians also teach us that healing is not simply the elimination of physical disease, but a process of reconnecting with our divine essence. Through meditative practices and channeling techniques, they guide us to access high vibrational frequencies that can transmute repressed emotions, limiting thought patterns, and energetic traumas. These teachings invite us to take responsibility for our well-being, recognizing that true healing begins within.

The relationship between Arcturians and human beings is based on mutual respect and free will. Unlike other belief systems or practices, Arcturian healing does not impose dogmas or require devotion. Instead, it presents itself as an accessible tool for those who wish to explore it, trusting in each individual's innate ability to discern and choose their own path.

The legacy of the Arcturians is also manifested in their ability to work with specific frequencies. These frequencies, which are often experienced as harmonic tones, vibrant colors, or sacred geometries, act as portals to expanded states of consciousness. Through these tools, the Arcturians invite us to explore higher dimensions and discover the vastness of our multidimensional being.

On the journey to healing, the Arcturians are not only guides, but also allies. Their energy is subtle, but deeply transformative, acting as a beacon that illuminates the path to our wholeness. Those who have worked with these frequencies describe experiences of profound clarity, inner peace, and a renewed sense of purpose.

However, it is important to remember that contact with the Arcturians is not exclusive to a few. It does not require extraordinary psychic abilities or special conditions. All that is needed is a genuine openness and a clear intention to connect with these higher energies. Through meditations, visualizations, and energy alignment practices, anyone can access this source of healing and wisdom.

Ultimately, the Arcturians do not seek adoration or recognition. Their purpose is simple, but profound: to help us remember our true nature as beings of light, capable of manifesting balance and harmony in all aspects of our existence. By opening ourselves to their guidance, we not only heal our wounds, but also awaken to the vast potential that resides within us.

The Arcturian presence is a reminder that we are not alone in our quest for healing and evolution. In the vast tapestry of the universe, we are part of an interconnected whole, and the Arcturians are here to support us every step of the way. As we continue to explore the teachings and practices that make up this healing system, their energy will continue to act as a beacon, guiding us to a life of greater balance, clarity, and purpose.

Chapter 2
Energy and Vibrational Anatomy

At the center of all that exists lies energy: an omnipresent, infinite, and constantly moving force. Although invisible to the physical eye, energy constitutes the foundation of the universe and permeates every corner of our existence. It is the subtle substance that connects the visible and invisible worlds, weaving a web that sustains and gives shape to life as we know it.

The principles of energy are universal and timeless. From the subatomic particles that vibrate in perfect harmony to the vast galaxies that spin in the cosmos, everything follows the laws of energy. This primordial essence has no beginning and no end; it simply flows and transforms, adapting to the myriad forms that make up reality.

In Arcturian healing, understanding the principles of energy is crucial to unraveling the mysteries of integral well-being. Vital energy, also known as prana, chi, or ki, is the flow that animates all living beings. It is the subtle breath that nourishes the physical, emotional, mental, and spiritual bodies, keeping them in balance. When this flow is free and harmonious, we experience health and vitality; when it is obstructed, imbalances arise that eventually manifest as illness or malaise.

Each human being is a microcosm within the universal macrocosm. In this interconnected system, our thoughts, emotions, and actions influence the flow of energy within us and around us. A positive thought generates a high vibration that extends to the surroundings, while dense emotions, such as fear or anger, can create energy blocks that interrupt the natural flow.

One of the fundamental concepts in this area is vibrational frequency. Everything in the universe has a specific vibration, from the densest stones to the brightest stars. In the case of human beings, our vibrational state is determined by a combination of factors, including our thoughts, emotions, and the general state of our energy body.

The highest frequencies, associated with emotions such as love, gratitude, and compassion, promote energy expansion and healing. On the other hand, the lower frequencies, related to emotions such as fear, hate, or sadness, tend to contract and obstruct the energy flow. This knowledge is the basis of many healing practices, including Arcturian healing, which seeks to raise the recipient's vibrational frequency to facilitate transformation.

Furthermore, energy is not static; it is in constant motion and interaction. Each person, object, and place has its own energetic imprint, which influences the surroundings and is influenced by it. This means that our interactions with other people and our immediate surroundings can have a significant impact on our energy state.

In the context of healing, energy acts as a bridge between the practitioner and the recipient. Through conscious intention, the practitioner can channel high frequencies to the recipient, helping them release blockages and restore natural flow. This process is not about imposing external energy, but about facilitating the recipient to realign with their own natural frequency.

Another essential principle is that of energy polarity. Just as in electricity, where there are positive and negative poles, energy also operates in polarities that must be kept in balance. The imbalance between these polarities can manifest as internal chaos, while their harmonization leads to a state of well-being.

In the human body, this principle is reflected in the interaction of various energies, such as masculine and feminine, active and passive, and those that connect with the elements of nature. Arcturian healing helps to restore this balance, promoting a complete integration of all parts of the being.

Energy interaction is not limited to individuals; it also occurs between us and the universe. Each thought and emotion we emit acts as a wave that travels through the universal energy field, interacting with other waves and creating resonance patterns. This phenomenon, known as the principle of vibrational correspondence, teaches us that we attract to ourselves what resonates with our vibration.

This has profound implications for healing, since consciously working with our energy allows us to change our vibration and, consequently, our experiences. For example, by releasing trapped emotions or negative mental patterns, we not only transform our internal state, but also open the door to new opportunities and connections more aligned with our purpose.

The Arcturians, as masters of energy, offer us tools and teachings that amplify our understanding of these principles. One of their most powerful legacies is the use of specific frequencies to tune and harmonize the human energy field. These frequencies, which are often experienced as sounds, colors, or subtle sensations, have the ability to penetrate deep into the being, promoting transformation on levels that transcend the physical.

For example, certain frequencies can dissolve emotional blockages accumulated over years, while others can raise the recipient's vibration, facilitating expanded states of consciousness. As we advance in our understanding of these principles, we learn to work with these frequencies in a conscious way, becoming co-creators of our healing and well-being.

Ultimately, the principles of energy invite us to rediscover our true nature as vibrational beings. They teach us that healing is not an isolated act, but a dynamic and continuous process of balance and expansion. By honoring these principles and applying them in our daily lives, we not only promote our own transformation, but also contribute to the balance and harmony of the universe as a whole.

Arcturian healing, with its focus on high frequencies and conscious intention, opens the door to a world of infinite possibilities, where each energy interaction becomes an opportunity to grow, heal, and transcend. With this knowledge, we are better equipped to enter the vast and fascinating world of energy anatomy, which we will explore in depth in the next steps of this journey.

The human body, so complex and fascinating in its biology, houses an even more subtle and equally intricate dimension: the energy system. This invisible web, composed of currents and energy centers, acts as the bridge between our physical form and the higher dimensions of our existence. Energy anatomy not only sustains life; it also reveals the secrets of our holistic well-being.

Each individual has a unique energy system that constantly interacts with the environment and cosmic forces. This system is made up of several interconnected elements: the chakras, the meridians, and the auric field. Together, they form a delicate ecosystem that profoundly influences our physical, emotional, mental, and spiritual health. Understanding this subtle network is fundamental to any healing practice, especially in the Arcturian system, which uses these structures as access points to transform and harmonize.

Chakras, a Sanskrit word meaning "wheel" or "vortex", are the primary energy centers of the human body. These swirling points act as gateways for energy, connecting our physical body with our subtle dimensions. Although there are many minor chakras, the Arcturian system focuses primarily on the seven main ones, which are aligned along the spine, from the base to the crown.

1. Root Chakra (Muladhara): Located at the base of the spine, this chakra is associated with security, stability, and our connection to the Earth. It is the foundation of our energy system, providing anchoring and support.
2. Sacral Chakra (Svadhisthana): Located just below the navel, this center governs emotions, creativity, and interpersonal relationships. It is a source of vital energy and emotional fluidity.
3. Solar Plexus Chakra (Manipura): Located in the stomach area, it represents personal power, confidence, and will. Here lies our capacity for action and determination.
4. Heart Chakra (Anahata): In the center of the chest, this chakra is the bridge between the physical and spiritual aspects. It is the epicenter of love, compassion, and connection with others.
5. Throat Chakra (Vishuddha): Located at the base of the throat, it governs communication and authentic expression. Here we channel our inner truth to the outside world.
6. Third Eye Chakra (Ajna): Between the eyebrows, this center is the gateway to intuition and spiritual perception. It facilitates vision beyond the physical and understanding of higher truths.
7. Crown Chakra (Sahasrara): At the top of the head, it connects with the higher dimensions and universal consciousness. It is the gateway to enlightenment and transcendence.

When the chakras are balanced, the flow of energy is harmonious and sustained, promoting health and clarity. However, blockages or imbalances in one or more chakras can manifest as physical illness, emotional conflict, or spiritual stagnation.

Meridians, on the other hand, are channels through which vital energy flows throughout the body. These energy pathways, widely recognized in Traditional Chinese Medicine, intersect and nourish organs and tissues, maintaining vitality. Just as arteries carry blood, meridians distribute energy to every cell, ensuring that the body functions in balance.

In the Arcturian system, meridians are seen as an essential network for connecting external and internal energies. Through specific practices, such as stimulation with Arcturian frequencies or guided visualization, these channels can be cleansed and revitalized, releasing blockages and optimizing energy flow.

The auric field, or aura, is the energy emanation that surrounds the physical body. This vibratory field acts as an extension of our essence, reflecting our inner state and protecting us from external influences. The densest layer of the aura is closely linked to the physical body, while the more subtle layers expand to higher dimensions, representing our emotional, mental, and spiritual aspects.

The aura is not only an indicator of our well-being; it is also a receiver and transmitter of energies. It constantly interacts with the environment, absorbing external influences and sending signals that reflect our vibrational frequency. A strong and balanced aura is essential to protect us from unwanted energies and maintain our connection to the universe.

In Arcturian healing, special attention is paid to cleansing and strengthening the auric field. Healing practices seek to repair any damage to this field, eliminate accumulated dense energies, and expand the luminosity of our aura. These techniques ensure that the recipient is fully aligned with the highest frequencies, promoting healing and transformation.

The human energy system also has an intimate relationship with the cosmos. Cosmic energies, from sources such as planets, stars, and higher dimensions, influence our energy field and, ultimately, our lives. The Arcturians, as high vibrational beings, understand this connection and use cosmic frequencies to work with our energy anatomy. Through these frequencies, they balance the chakras, unblock the meridians, and strengthen the aura, restoring integral balance.

Energy anatomy is a direct reflection of our health and well-being. Each blockage, each imbalance, and each distortion in this system has its origin in our experiences, thoughts, and emotions. By addressing these roots through healing practices, we not only restore energy flow, but also create the conditions for lasting well-being.

Chapter 3
Preparation and Holistic Healing

Before accessing the high frequencies of healing and transformation that the Arcturians offer, it is essential to prepare the inner ground: our spiritual and mental being. This process not only allows us to receive and channel the energies more effectively, but also strengthens our connection to the higher levels of consciousness. Spiritual preparation is not an externally imposed requirement, but an invitation to align ourselves with the purity and clarity necessary to work with these subtle and powerful forces.

At the heart of this preparation lies conscious intention. Through it, we direct our mind and spirit towards a clear purpose: to open ourselves to healing and Arcturian energies. This intention acts as a vibrational key that attunes our frequency to the higher dimensions, allowing energies to flow freely and without obstruction.

One of the fundamental pillars in this process is the practice of meditation. Meditation is not simply an act of relaxation, but a profound method for calming the mind, stilling external distractions, and centering attention on our inner core. It is in this state of calm and receptivity that the bridge between the physical and the spiritual is established, an open channel through which Arcturian frequencies can manifest.

- 1. Meditation as an energetic anchor

To begin, it is essential to create a sacred space, an environment that invites introspection and stillness. This space can be a quiet corner of the house, decorated with symbolic elements such as crystals, candles, or images that resonate with the energy of peace and connection. More importantly, the environment should reflect a clear intention of respect and spiritual focus.

Once the environment is established, the practitioner can adopt a comfortable posture, preferably sitting with the spine straight, to facilitate the flow of energy. Closing the eyes helps to disconnect from the external world and direct attention inwards. This is where the alignment process begins, allowing the breath to become a subtle guide to a state of deep relaxation.

Conscious breathing is a key component in spiritual preparation. Inhaling deeply while visualizing the entry of pure light and exhaling releasing any tension or worry allows the body and mind to enter a state of balance. This breathing rhythm, combined with the visualization of light, acts as an energetic magnet, attracting the high frequencies necessary for healing practice.

- 2. Grounding: the art of balancing the subtle and the tangible

Before ascending to the higher dimensions, it is essential to establish a firm connection with the Earth. This process, known as grounding, ensures that our physical body remains balanced as we explore the more ethereal energies. Without this connection, we could feel disoriented, scattered, or even overwhelmed by the intensity of the higher frequencies.

A simple exercise to achieve this connection is to visualize roots emerging from the soles of the feet, penetrating deep into the ground. These roots symbolize our union with Earth's energy, allowing us to draw stability and strength from the planet's core. During this exercise, one can mentally repeat an affirmation such as, "I am anchored and balanced, connected to the energy of the Earth."

- 3. Purification as inner preparation

Another crucial step in spiritual preparation is energy cleansing. This process involves releasing the dense or stagnant energies that can accumulate in our auric field and energy system. These energies can come from our daily interactions, unprocessed negative emotions, or external influences.

Purification can be carried out through various practices, such as the use of crystals, baths with mineral salts, or the burning of herbs such as incense or sage. In addition, visualization is a powerful tool: imagining a cascade of white light flowing through our body, cleansing and renewing every cell and every fiber of our being, is a simple but profoundly effective technique.

- 4. The role of intention and devotion

In Arcturian healing, intention is not just a thought or desire, but an active vibration that shapes energy and directs it toward a purpose. Before any practice, it is essential to state the intention clearly, either silently or aloud. For example, a common affirmation could be: "I open myself to receive the Arcturian healing energies with love and gratitude, for my highest good and the good of all beings."

Along with intention, devotion to practice is what creates a stable and receptive energy channel. This is not about devotion in a religious sense, but about a sincere and constant commitment to personal development and connection with higher energies.

- 5. The proper mental state

Mental state plays a crucial role in spiritual preparation. Cultivating a calm, receptive, and non-judgmental mind creates the ideal space for Arcturian frequencies to fully integrate. Although the human mind tends to wander and generate intrusive thoughts, the regular practice of meditation and conscious breathing can help us redirect our attention to the present moment.

The Arcturians teach us that trust is an essential quality during this process. Trusting in our abilities, in the guidance of these beings, and in the natural flow of energy allows us to let go of resistance and fully open ourselves to the healing experience.

- 6. Preliminary practices with Arcturian frequencies

For those beginning to explore Arcturian energies, it may be helpful to work with specific frequencies before approaching advanced practices. These frequencies, often experienced as subtle tones or vibrations, help to attune the energy system to the higher dimensions.

An initial practice is to listen to high vibrational music or binaural beats designed to activate spiritual connection. During this experience, the practitioner can visualize a ray of blue or violet light descending from the cosmos to their crown, filling every cell with renewing energy.

- 7. Culmination of preparation

Spiritual preparation is not a one-time event, but an ongoing practice that strengthens our energy system and aligns us with our higher purpose. By adopting these practices regularly, we create fertile ground for Arcturian energies to manifest in their full magnitude.

Over time, this process not only empowers us to channel and receive these energies, but also profoundly transforms our relationship with ourselves, with the universe, and with the purpose of healing. It is from this state of alignment that we are ready to explore the broader and deeper aspects of the Arcturian holistic healing system.

In the vastness of the universe, where each atom is intrinsically connected to the next, a profound truth unfolds: existence is an interdependent dance between the physical, the emotional, the mental, and the spiritual. The Arcturian holistic healing system reflects this truth, offering a perspective that transcends the limitations of linear thinking. Instead of seeing the human being as a set of separate parts, this approach considers it as an integrated whole, where each aspect influences and is influenced by the others.

The holistic system is not a new idea, but a high vibrational reinterpretation that the Arcturians have developed to align with humanity's evolutionary needs. At its core, this system recognizes that true healing is not simply the absence of disease, but the dynamic balance that sustains well-being at all levels of being.

- 8. The Arcturian vision of energetic interdependence

From the Arcturian perspective, the universe is a unified field of energy, where each element is part of a vibrational web. The human being is no exception: our bodies, emotions, thoughts and spirit are expressions of the same energetic source. This view implies that any imbalance in one area inevitably affects the others.

For example, an unresolved emotional trauma can manifest as a physical illness, while negative mental patterns can block spiritual connection. Similarly, spiritual well-being can raise the energy of the physical body and foster more balanced emotions. The holistic system is based on this interconnection, addressing the individual as a whole, rather than focusing on isolated symptoms.

- 9. The pillars of the Arcturian holistic system

The Arcturian holistic approach rests on four main pillars, each representing an essential aspect of the human being:

- 10. Physical body: It is the tangible vehicle that allows us to interact with the material world. The Arcturians teach that the physical body must be nurtured and respected as a sacred temple. Healing practices include not only energy harmonization, but also conscious care of the

body through nutrition, rest, and balanced physical activity.
- 11. Emotions: Emotions are energy in motion, and their free flow is vital for well-being. Arcturian energies are used to release emotional blockages, transmute patterns of fear and pain, and cultivate states of love, gratitude, and compassion.
- 12. Mind: The mind is a powerful tool, capable of creating both positive and limiting realities. The Arcturian holistic system teaches practices to reprogram negative thoughts and raise mental frequency, which facilitates a clearer and more expansive perception.
- 13. Spirit: This is the core of being, the divine spark that connects the individual with the universal source. Arcturian healing strengthens this connection, helping people to remember their divine essence and their highest purpose.
- 14. The integration of the levels of being

The Arcturian holistic system does not address these levels in isolation. Instead, it seeks to integrate them into a harmonious flow. For example, a practice may begin with the relaxation of the physical body through conscious breathing, followed by the release of trapped emotions through visualizations, and culminating in a deep connection with spiritual energy. This multidimensional approach ensures that healing is complete and lasting.
- 15. Tools of the Arcturian holistic system

The Arcturians have developed a unique set of tools and techniques that amplify the effectiveness of the holistic system. These tools are not external, but vibrational, designed to interact directly with human energy fields.

- High frequencies: Arcturian frequencies are subtle energies that vibrate in resonance with the higher dimensions. Through these frequencies, it is possible to cleanse, balance and strengthen the energy field, allowing vital energy to flow without obstruction.
- Sacred geometry: Geometric patterns have the ability to influence energy in specific ways. The Arcturians use shapes such as the star tetrahedron, the golden spiral, and Metatron's cube to restore harmony and amplify spiritual connection.
- Conscious intention: Intention is a creative force that directs energy toward a specific purpose. In the Arcturian holistic system, intention is used to program frequencies and sacred geometries, enhancing their impact.
- Guided visualization: This technique helps the mind to focus and create an internal environment conducive to healing. Visualizations may include the perception of purifying light, the expansion of the aura, or connection with spiritual guides.
- 16. Healing as a co-creation process

The Arcturian holistic system teaches that healing is not something that is imposed from the outside, but a process of co-creation between the practitioner and the recipient. The Arcturians, in their role as guides, facilitate access to higher energies, but the recipient is the active agent who integrates and uses these energies for their transformation.

This approach fosters personal responsibility, encouraging each individual to take an active role in their well-being. By recognizing and working with internal imbalances, the recipient not only experiences healing, but also develops a greater awareness of themselves and their ability to maintain balance.

- 17. Practical applications of the holistic system

The Arcturian holistic system has broad applications ranging from self-healing to working with others. Some of the practices include:
- Harmonization of the chakras: Using frequencies and visualizations to balance energy centers.
- Emotional release: Working with specific frequencies to dissolve emotional blockages and promote inner clarity.
- Guided meditation: Designed to align body, mind and spirit with higher energies.
- Distance healing: Applying Arcturian techniques to help others, regardless of their physical location.
- 18. The profound impact of the holistic system

As the Arcturian holistic system is integrated into daily life, it not only transforms the individual, but also positively impacts their environment. Personal healing creates waves that extend to others, contributing to collective and planetary balance.

The Arcturians remind us that this system is not an end in itself, but a path to reconnection with our divine essence. By applying its principles, we not only heal our wounds, but also awaken to our innate capacity to live in balance and fullness.

This is the power of the holistic system: a tool for personal transformation that resonates with the highest vibrations of the universe, guiding us to a harmonious and fulfilling existence at all levels of being.

Chapter 4
Frequencies and Creative Power

At the heart of Arcturian healing lies a fundamental principle: everything in the universe vibrates. From the smallest particle to the vastest galaxies, every aspect of existence is in constant motion, emitting and resonating with specific frequencies. These vibrations not only determine the nature of matter, but also influence our physical, emotional, mental, and spiritual experience.

Arcturian frequencies are unique vibrations originating from higher dimensions, designed to interact with human energy systems and facilitate healing, balance, and transformation. These frequencies, channeled by the Arcturians, act as a bridge between the earthly and the cosmic, helping us access higher states of consciousness and release deep blockages that limit our evolution.

1. The Nature of Arcturian Frequencies

Unlike the frequencies we perceive with our physical senses, such as sound or visible light, Arcturian frequencies operate at more subtle vibrational levels. These energies are not restricted by the limitations of time and space, allowing them to interact directly with our energy anatomy, even at great distances.

Each Arcturian frequency carries a specific intention and is designed to address particular aspects of being. Some are focused on cleansing and releasing energy blocks, while others promote vibrational elevation, spiritual connection, or deep healing of emotional and physical traumas.

2. The Vibrational Language of the Universe

The Arcturians teach that these frequencies are a universal language that transcends words and concepts. This vibrational language communicates directly with our cells, tissues, and energy systems, carrying information that activates healing and transformation processes.

When we work with these frequencies, we are inviting our being to realign with its natural state of balance. As our internal vibrations adjust to the Arcturian frequencies, a resonance phenomenon occurs that dissolves discordant energies and restores harmony.

3. How We Perceive Arcturian Frequencies

Although these frequencies are not always audible or visible, many people experience them in subtle yet significant ways. Some describe physical sensations, such as gentle warmth, tingling, or slight pressure in specific areas of the body. Others perceive colors, geometric patterns, or ethereal sounds during connection practices.

These experiences are the result of the interaction between Arcturian frequencies and our energy fields. However, it is not necessary to "feel" something to benefit from these energies. Their impact is profound and manifests on multiple levels, even if we are not aware of it at the time.

4. Channeling Arcturian Frequencies

Arcturian healing practitioners act as channels for these frequencies, allowing them to flow through them to the recipients. This process does not require effort, but rather a conscious openness and a clear intention to serve as an energy bridge.

Preparing to channel these frequencies involves practices such as meditation, energy purification, and establishing an intention aligned with the well-being of the recipient. Once in this receptive state, the practitioner simply becomes a vehicle for the Arcturian frequencies to do their work.

5. Applications of Arcturian Frequencies

Arcturian frequencies can be employed in a wide variety of contexts and for diverse purposes. Some of their most common applications include:

6. Energy cleansing: These frequencies are particularly effective in dissolving dense energies and releasing blockages that obstruct the natural flow of vital energy.
7. Chakra balancing: Specific frequencies can tune each chakra, restoring its ideal vibration and facilitating the harmonious flow of energy throughout the body.
8. Emotional healing: Many of these vibrations are designed to deal with trapped emotions, such as fear, sadness, or anger, helping to release and

transmute them into higher states of love and peace.
9. Spiritual connection: By raising the overall vibration of the recipient, these frequencies facilitate the opening of the higher channels of consciousness, strengthening the connection with the higher self and the spiritual dimensions.
10. Physical healing: Although they work primarily on energetic levels, these frequencies can have a profound impact on the physical body, accelerating recovery and promoting cell regeneration.
11. Techniques for Working with Arcturian Frequencies

The use of these frequencies is not limited to advanced practitioners; anyone can learn to connect with them and benefit from their transformative power. The following are some simple but effective techniques:
1. Meditation with frequencies: During meditation, the practitioner can visualize a beam of vibrant light descending from the cosmos, carrying the Arcturian frequencies into their body and filling it with renewing energy.
2. Listening to vibrational tones or music: Many practitioners use recordings that replicate Arcturian frequencies to create a resonant environment. These recordings act as a portal to higher dimensions, facilitating connection.
3. Laying on of hands: In this practice, the practitioner places their hands on the recipient's

body, allowing the frequencies to flow through them into the recipient's energy field.
4. Use of sacred geometry: Geometric shapes associated with Arcturian frequencies can be visualized or physically represented to amplify healing.

12. The Profound Impact of Frequencies

Working with Arcturian frequencies not only transforms the individual, but also has a ripple effect on their surroundings. When a person raises their vibration, they contribute to the collective balance, radiating harmonious energy to those around them.

This impact is not limited to the human level; Arcturian frequencies can also be used to heal spaces, harmonize relationships, and contribute to planetary well-being. The Arcturians consider this expansive application to be an essential aspect of their mission, helping humanity not only to heal, but to evolve into a state of conscious unity.

Arcturian frequencies are more than just vibrations; they are the direct manifestation of a cosmic intelligence that seeks to balance and elevate all beings. As we learn to work with these energies, we not only transform our lives, but also align ourselves with the highest purpose of our existence: to be conscious co-creators of a more harmonious world.

From this point, the journey towards mastery in Arcturian healing continues, deepening the understanding and application of these frequencies to unlock the vast potential that resides within each being.

In the subtle interweaving of the universe, where every thought, emotion, and action has an echo, intention rises as a primordial force. Beyond the visible, beyond words, intention is the beacon that guides energy to its purpose. In the context of Arcturian healing, this principle acquires central relevance, for it is intention that directs, focuses, and amplifies the high frequencies, transforming them into tools of profound healing and transformation.

Intention is more than just a wish or a thought. It is an active vibration, a conscious impulse that acts as a catalyst in the healing process. The moment a clear intention is established, the universe begins to reconfigure itself to align with that guideline. It is as if every cell, every atom, responds to this vibrational signal, facilitating the flow of energy towards the desired goal.

In Arcturian practice, intention becomes the key that opens the door to higher dimensions. The Arcturians, when working with their high frequencies, respond directly to the clarity and purity of the intentions of those who seek to connect with them. Without a defined intention, energy can be dispersed, diluting its impact. But with a focused intention, the frequencies find a clear channel to manifest, creating a vibrational bridge between the practitioner and the higher dimensions.

Consciously directing energy begins with a deep understanding of what one wishes to achieve. Before starting any healing practice, it is essential to take a moment to reflect and connect with the purpose behind the action. It is not simply a matter of formulating a sentence, but of feeling it, of imbuing it with emotion and conviction. For example, an intention such as "releasing energy blocks to promote harmony in my life" should resonate deeply within the practitioner, creating an emotional connection that enhances its vibration.

Intention not only defines the purpose, but also acts as a guide for energy. Instead of flowing randomly, energy aligns with the vibration of intention, moving to where it is most needed. This principle is especially important in Arcturian healing, where high frequencies can address multiple levels of being. A clear intention ensures that energy is used efficiently, maximizing its impact on the recipient.

Focus and full presence are essential to strengthen intention. In a world full of distractions, it is easy to allow the mind to wander, weakening the clarity of intention. During practice, the practitioner must be fully present, preventing intrusive thoughts from interfering with the flow of energy. This presence does not require perfection, but rather a conscious commitment to return to the present moment whenever the mind deviates.

Intention not only influences the direction of energy, but also its quality. An intention based on high emotions, such as love, compassion, and gratitude, generates a higher vibration, which in turn amplifies the impact of Arcturian frequencies. On the other hand, an intention motivated by fear, anger, or selfishness can create an energetic distortion, limiting its effectiveness. Therefore, the Arcturians emphasize the importance of purifying the heart and mind before setting any intention.

Intention is not only a tool for directing energy to the recipient, but also a means to create a transformative space. By establishing an intention, the practitioner declares their willingness to open up to healing, trust the process, and allow the Arcturian frequencies to do their work. This act of openness and surrender is fundamental, as it removes internal barriers that could block the flow of energy.

The importance of intention also extends beyond the context of healing. In everyday life, every thought and action is imbued with an intention, conscious or unconscious. By becoming more aware of these intentions, the individual can begin to shape their reality in a way that is more aligned with their values and purposes. The Arcturians teach that intention is not an isolated event, but a continuous flow that permeates every aspect of existence.

The impact of intention is magnified when combined with other tools of the Arcturian holistic system, such as visualizations, frequencies, and sacred geometry. For example, when working with a geometric pattern, intention can program the vibration of that symbol, directing it towards a specific purpose. Similarly, when visualizing a ray of light flowing into an area of the body, intention focuses and amplifies the energy, accelerating the healing process.

Although intention is a powerful tool, it requires practice and refinement. It is not always easy to maintain a clear intention, especially when the mind is full of distractions or conflicting emotions. However, with patience and dedication, the practitioner can develop the ability to establish increasingly precise and effective intentions.

The Arcturians, as guides, are always willing to support this process. By working with them, one can ask for guidance to clarify intentions and ensure that they are aligned with the greater good. This collaboration not only strengthens the connection with Arcturian frequencies, but also promotes a sense of trust and empowerment in the practitioner.

In the end, intention is more than a technique; it is an expression of the very essence of being. It is the spark that initiates the healing process, the force that transforms energy, and the thread that connects the individual to the universe. By mastering intention, the practitioner not only becomes a channel for Arcturian frequencies, but also a conscious co-creator of their own reality, capable of manifesting harmony, balance, and healing at all levels of their existence.

Chapter 5
Connection and Sacred Tools

The universe is woven by a vast network of energies, and within this infinite flow, human beings possess the innate ability to establish deep connections with higher frequencies. Arcturian energies, with their elevated and transformative vibration, are always present, waiting for the conscious seeker to extend their intention and align with them. Connection techniques are bridges that allow us to open ourselves to these energies, channel them, and harness their healing power.

Connecting with Arcturian frequencies does not require extraordinary abilities or unattainable mystical gifts. It is an act of alignment and openness that combines intention, focus, and specific practices. Through these techniques, anyone can experience the flow of these energies, whether for personal healing or to facilitate healing in others.

The first step towards this connection is to establish a space of receptivity. This space does not only refer to the physical environment, but also to the practitioner's inner state. Creating a peaceful environment free from distractions helps the mind and body enter a relaxed state, conducive to energetic connection. A place dedicated exclusively to these practices, decorated with symbolic elements such as crystals, candles, or sacred geometry, can amplify intention and foster a sense of sacredness.

Conscious breathing is an essential tool in these practices. Through breathing, we not only calm the mind but also activate the flow of energy in our body. An effective technique consists of inhaling deeply, imagining that pure light is being absorbed from the cosmos, and exhaling while visualizing the release of any tension or blockage. This constant rhythm of breathing creates a vibrational bridge that connects the physical body with the higher dimensions.

One of the fundamental techniques for connecting with Arcturian energies is guided visualization. In this process, the practitioner uses their mind to imagine a flow of energy that surrounds and penetrates them. A common exercise consists of visualizing a ray of blue or violet light descending from the stars towards the crown of the head, entering the body and filling it with a sense of peace and renewal. This light is not merely imagined; it is a vibrational representation of the Arcturian frequencies, which respond directly to the practitioner's intention.

Meditation is another essential practice for establishing and deepening this connection. During meditation, the practitioner seeks to silence superficial thoughts and open themselves to universal energy. An effective method is to sit in a comfortable posture, with the back straight, and concentrate on the flow of breath. As the mind calms down, one can focus on a mantra or affirmation, such as "I am open to the Arcturian healing frequencies", repeating it with each breath. The repetition of the mantra, combined with clear intention, creates a vibrational field that resonates with Arcturian frequencies, facilitating their access. This approach not only promotes connection but also strengthens the practitioner's confidence in their ability to channel these energies.

Another powerful technique is the use of sound as a connection tool. The Arcturians, when working with specific frequencies, recognize the power of sound to alter states of consciousness and open portals to higher dimensions. Listening to binaural beats, vibrational music, or sounds created with instruments such as Tibetan bowls or tuning forks can amplify the practitioner's ability to tune into Arcturian energies.

The body also plays a crucial role in these practices. Gentle and conscious movements, such as those found in disciplines like yoga or tai chi chuan, can help open energy channels and prepare the system to receive high frequencies. These movements, combined with breathing and visualization, foster a state of total alignment.

As the practitioner becomes familiar with these techniques, they may begin to experience subtle sensations that indicate a successful connection. These sensations may include a gentle warmth in certain areas of the body, an inner vibration, or a feeling of expansion and lightness. Although these experiences vary from person to person, they all reflect the interaction between the human energy system and Arcturian frequencies.

For those seeking to further deepen the connection, working with specific crystals can be of great help. Crystals such as quartz, amethyst, or selenite have vibrational properties that resonate with Arcturian energies. Placing these crystals near the body, holding them in the hands during meditation, or using them in sacred geometry patterns amplifies the energy field and facilitates attunement with these frequencies.

Time and patience are essential elements in the development of these practices. Connecting with Arcturian frequencies does not always occur immediately or spectacularly. Often, it is a gradual process that requires consistency and dedication. Each practice session reinforces the practitioner's ability to open up and receive these energies, leading to increasingly deeper experiences.

The Arcturians, in their wisdom and compassion, emphasize that connection is not a privilege reserved for a few. It is available to all those who are willing to explore their energetic potential and open themselves to transformation. Through regular practice and conscious intention, anyone can become a channel for these frequencies, experiencing not only their healing power but also a deep connection with the higher dimensions of the universe.

Connecting with Arcturian energies is a journey of integration and expansion. By learning these techniques and applying them in daily life, the practitioner not only develops their ability to channel energies but also transforms their relationship with the universe and themselves. Opening to these frequencies is the beginning of a path of discovery and healing that continues to reveal new possibilities with every step.

Access to Arcturian frequencies and the unfolding of their transformative power are enhanced by a set of tools and resources that act as catalysts and amplifiers of healing practices. These tools, although seemingly simple, are imbued with deep energetic significance, capable of resonating with higher dimensions and creating a bridge between the tangible and the subtle. Each is designed to facilitate the connection, channeling, and integration of Arcturian energies, allowing the practitioner to deepen their experience and optimize their healing work.

Sacred geometry is one of the most fundamental tools within the Arcturian system. These forms, such as Metatron's Cube, the Flower of Life, and the Merkaba, are not mere figures, but vibrational representations of universal patterns that sustain creation. By working with these geometries, whether through meditations, visualizations, or physical representations, the practitioner can align their energy with the harmonic principles of the cosmos. These forms act as portals to higher dimensions, channeling frequencies that cleanse, balance, and strengthen the human energy field.

Crystals are another powerful resource in Arcturian healing. Each crystal has a unique frequency that interacts with the user's energy system, amplifying and modulating the energies that flow through it. Crystals such as clear quartz, which acts as a universal amplifier, or amethyst, known for its purifying and spiritual connection properties, are especially useful in these practices. By placing crystals on the chakras, holding them in the hands during meditation, or using them in geometric patterns, the practitioner can intensify their connection with Arcturian frequencies and enhance their healing effect.

Sound and vibration are essential tools for accessing and working with Arcturian frequencies. Specific tones, binaural frequencies, and instruments such as Tibetan bowls and gongs generate sound waves that resonate with the energy system, helping to release blockages and raise vibration. The Arcturians, known for their affinity with sound, often transmit frequencies through ethereal tones that practitioners can perceive in meditative states. Listening to high vibrational music or chanting specific mantras can also facilitate alignment with these energies.

Light and color are other fundamental tools within this system. Each color has a unique frequency that interacts with the human energy field in a specific way. For example, blue, associated with tranquility and communication, can be used to balance the throat chakra, while violet, connected with transmutation and spirituality, is ideal for working with the crown chakra. Visualizing lights of specific colors flowing to areas of the body, or using lamps and color filters during practices, can amplify the connection with Arcturian energies.

The conscious use of intention is also a powerful tool. Intention does not require any external object, but its impact is profound and transformative. By setting a clear intention before each practice, the practitioner directs energy toward a specific purpose, optimizing its flow and effectiveness. This intention can be reinforced using affirmations such as: "I am open to receiving and channeling Arcturian energies for my highest good and the good of all beings." These affirmations act as vibrational anchors that focus and align the energy system with the desired purpose.

The practitioner's hands, as direct extensions of the human energy system, are natural tools of great power. The laying on of hands is an ancient practice that finds a central place in Arcturian healing. By placing the hands on or near the recipient's body, the practitioner allows energies to flow through them into the recipient's energy field, facilitating cleansing, balancing, and regeneration.

The environment in which healing practices take place also plays an important role. A sacred, clean, and orderly space can amplify the connection with Arcturian frequencies. Elements such as candles, incense, symbolic images, and ambient music help create an environment conducive to introspection and receptivity. Dedicating a specific place for these practices can strengthen the practitioner's intention and establish a stable energy field that facilitates connection.

Water, as a conductor of energy, is an often underestimated but extremely useful resource in healing. The Arcturians teach that water can be programmed with specific intentions and frequencies to amplify its impact on the body and spirit. By holding a container of water while visualizing healing energies flowing into it, the practitioner can create a vibrational tool that, when drunk, works directly with the internal energy system.

Writing and symbols also have a place within Arcturian tools. Arcturian symbols, channeled by experienced practitioners, contain vibrational patterns that resonate with specific frequencies. Drawing these symbols, whether on paper or visualizing them in the air, can serve to activate certain aspects of the energy system or to direct energy toward a particular purpose.

Time and patience are fundamental resources that are often overlooked. Connecting with Arcturian energies, although accessible, may take time for the practitioner to develop a keener sensitivity and greater channeling capacity. Dedicating time regularly to practices strengthens the connection and allows for a deeper integration of frequencies into the practitioner's energy system.

These tools and resources are not ends in themselves, but rather means to facilitate connection, focus, and amplification of Arcturian energies. It is not necessary to use them all at once, nor to rely solely on them. The most important thing is that the practitioner develops a personal and conscious relationship with each tool, discovering which ones resonate most deeply with their energy system and purpose.

As the practitioner becomes familiar with these tools, their ability to work with Arcturian frequencies expands, allowing them to address more complex challenges and achieve deeper levels of healing. These tools, combined with clear intention and constant dedication, transform the practice of healing into a vibrational art that not only benefits the recipient but also elevates the practitioner to new dimensions of consciousness and mastery.

Chapter 6
Connection and Sacred Tools

Healing, in its purest essence, is a natural and continuous process that seeks to restore balance in all levels of being. Although often perceived as a complex act reserved for advanced practitioners, the fundamentals of healing are accessible to all. The Arcturians remind us that the power to heal is intrinsically linked to our connection with universal energy, an omnipresent force that flows through us and around us, waiting to be activated by a clear and conscious intention.

On the path to healing, it is essential to understand that each human being is a channel of energy. This channel can be obstructed by emotional blockages, limiting mental patterns or accumulated stress. Simple healing practices seek to release these obstructions and restore the natural flow of vital energy. The first step towards this goal is to recognize the intimate relationship between the physical body and the energy system, understanding that any imbalance in one inevitably affects the other.

One of the basic principles of healing is energy alignment. This process involves balancing the body's energy centers and channels, allowing the life force to flow without restriction. Although alignment may seem like an abstract concept, it manifests in concrete physical and emotional sensations, such as greater vitality, mental clarity and emotional stability.

Conscious breathing is a fundamental tool to initiate this process. Each inhalation and exhalation act as vehicles for the flow of energy, helping to release accumulated tensions and establish a state of receptive calm. A basic technique consists of sitting in a comfortable posture, closing your eyes and concentrating on your breathing, inhaling deeply through your nose while visualizing pure light filling your body, and exhaling through your mouth while releasing any feeling of heaviness or blockage. This simple exercise can be performed anytime, anywhere, providing immediate anchoring to the present and renewed access to universal energy.

In addition to breathing, the use of hands as energy channels is a central practice in the fundamentals of healing. The hands, being directly connected to the energy centers of the heart and mind, act as bridges between the practitioner and the receiver of energy. A common practice is the laying on of hands, where the practitioner places the palms on or near the recipient's body, allowing energy to flow to the areas that need it most.

The key to this technique lies not in strength or effort, but in clear intention and a state of surrender. The practitioner does not "give" energy from their own system, but acts as a channel for universal frequencies.

Before beginning, it is helpful to set an intention, such as "I allow energy to flow freely for the greater good." This simple statement creates an open and receptive energy space, optimizing the impact of the practice.

Visualization also plays an important role in the fundamentals of healing. Through the mind, the practitioner can direct energy to specific areas of the body or energy field. For example, by visualizing a golden light flowing to the heart area, one can release accumulated emotional tension and restore harmony to this vital center.

A basic visualization technique consists of imagining a ray of light descending from the cosmos, entering through the crown of the head and flowing down, clearing each chakra and filling the body with renewing energy. This practice not only helps to release blockages, but also strengthens the practitioner's energy field, creating a natural barrier against negative external influences.

Regular repetition of these basic practices is essential to build a solid foundation in healing. Consistency allows the practitioner to develop greater sensitivity to subtle energies, learning to recognize changes in their own energy field and that of others. Although results may vary from day to day, each session contributes to the development of a deeper connection with universal energy.

In addition to individual practices, the environment plays an important role in the healing process. A clean, tidy and positively charged space can amplify the effectiveness of practices. Elements such as crystals, candles or soft music can be used to create a conducive environment, but the most important thing is the energy that the practitioner brings to the space.

Respect for the process is another key aspect of the fundamentals of healing. Healing is not always an immediate event; it is often a gradual journey that requires patience and self-compassion. The Arcturians teach that every practice, no matter how small, contributes to the overall balance of the energy system. Even seemingly insignificant efforts, such as a few minutes of conscious breathing a day, can have a significant cumulative impact.

It is important to remember that the fundamentals of healing are not an end in themselves, but a preparation for more advanced practices. These basic techniques establish fertile ground from which the practitioner can explore deeper dimensions of Arcturian healing. By mastering these simple tools, one develops confidence in the innate human capacity to heal, laying the foundation for working with higher and more complex frequencies in the future.

Healing is a process of continuous transformation. Each practice, each breath and each intention are steps on a path to harmony and integral well-being. Through these fundamentals, the practitioner not only learns to release blockages and restore balance, but also to recognize their connection to a greater universal force. In this recognition lies the true power of healing: the ability to transform not only the body, but also the mind, the spirit and, ultimately, life itself.

Breathing, an action so natural that it often goes unnoticed, is actually one of the most powerful tools in the art of healing. In each inhalation and exhalation resides a flow of vital energy that connects the physical body with the spiritual dimensions. The Arcturians teach that breathing not only sustains physical life, but also acts as a vibrational bridge between the different levels of being, allowing harmonization and healing through conscious access to its power.

Conscious breathing raises the vibration and stabilizes the energy system. When performed in a deliberate and rhythmic manner, it promotes the expansion of vital energy, releasing blockages and facilitating the flow of higher frequencies through the body. It is the foundation upon which many of the Arcturian healing practices are built, as it provides solid grounding while allowing connection to higher energies.

One of the simplest, yet most effective, ways to work with the breath is the technique known as conscious deep breathing. In this practice, the practitioner inhales slowly and deeply through the nose, allowing the air to completely fill the lungs, and then exhales in a controlled manner through the mouth. Meanwhile, visualize pure light entering with each inhalation and any tension or stagnant energy leaving with each exhalation. This process not only calms the mind, but also cleanses the energy system, preparing the body to receive higher frequencies.

In addition to deep breathing, there is the technique of cyclical breathing, in which the practitioner maintains a constant flow without pauses between inhalation and exhalation. This technique creates a state of energy flow that activates the subtle centers and amplifies access to Arcturian frequencies. During this practice, many feel a slight vibration in the body or a sense of expansion, indicating that energies are beginning to flow more freely.

Another common practice is chakra-focused breathing. In this technique, the practitioner directs their attention to a specific chakra while breathing, visualizing energy flowing to and activating that center. For example, when working with the heart chakra, the practitioner can imagine a green or pink light expanding with each inhalation, filling the area with love and compassion, and clearing any emotional blockage with each exhalation.

Breathing can also be used to connect with Arcturian frequencies more directly. An advanced technique consists of visualizing a ray of light descending from the higher dimensions to the crown of the head while inhaling, allowing this energy to flow through the body with each breath. This process can be intensified by incorporating vocal sounds such as "om" or specific tones that resonate with Arcturian frequencies, helping to attune the energy system to these higher vibrations.

The rhythm and cadence of breathing also have a significant impact on the practitioner's vibrational state. Rapid, shallow breaths tend to contract the energy system, while deep, slow breaths expand it. The Arcturians teach that by deliberately slowing down the breath, the practitioner not only calms the body and mind, but also attunes to the natural flow of universal energy, facilitating connection to higher frequencies.

The practice of breath retention, known as kumbhaka in certain traditions, is another powerful technique that can be adapted to the Arcturian healing system. In this practice, the practitioner inhales deeply, holds the breath for a few seconds while visualizing energy concentrating in a specific area, and then exhales in a controlled manner. This approach allows for deeper work with energy, intensifying its effect on the physical and subtle body.

Breathing not only facilitates connection to higher energies, but also acts as a regulator of the nervous system and an emotional stabilizer. During times of stress or imbalance, the practice of conscious breathing can be used to restore balance, calming the mind and heart. This regulating effect is especially useful before performing any healing practice, as it ensures that the practitioner is in an ideal state of receptivity.

The importance of breathing extends beyond individual practices. In healing sessions with others, the rhythm and intention behind the practitioner's breathing can influence the recipient's energy field. For example, by attuning the breath to that of the recipient, the practitioner creates a resonant field that facilitates energy transfer and amplifies the impact of healing.

The Arcturians also emphasize the role of breathing in integrating higher energies. Often, after working with high frequencies, the energy system needs time to assimilate and balance these new vibrations. During this process, conscious breathing acts as an anchor, helping to stabilize energy and avoid possible symptoms of overload, such as dizziness or fatigue.

In everyday life, breathing can be a constant tool for maintaining balance and spiritual connection. Through brief but intentional moments of conscious breathing, the practitioner can re-center, release accumulated tension and renew their energy flow. These regular pauses not only promote well-being, but also strengthen the practitioner's ability to work with more advanced energies in the future.

Breathing is, ultimately, much more than a physiological act. It is an expression of the universal flow that connects all beings with the source of life. By learning to use it consciously, the practitioner not only transforms their healing experience, but also deepens their connection to the higher dimensions and their own divine essence. This simple, yet powerful resource reminds us that healing is not in something external, but in our innate ability to work with the tools we already possess, and breathing is undoubtedly one of the most essential and transformative.

Chapter 7
Ethics and Energy Purification

The practice of healing is a profoundly sacred act that requires not only skills and knowledge but also a solid ethical commitment. In the Arcturian holistic healing system, ethics is not a complement, but the foundation upon which all practice is built. The Arcturians, as high-vibrational guides, emphasize that the energy we channel and direct must be used with respect, compassion, and an intention aligned with the highest good of all beings involved.

The practitioner's responsibility is one of the fundamental pillars in the ethics of healing. This commitment implies a conscious recognition that working with subtle energies has a profound impact on the recipient's energy system and, in some cases, on their life in general. Therefore, the practitioner must approach each session with an attitude of respect and humility, understanding that they are facilitating a process that belongs to the recipient and not to themselves.

Respect for free will is another central principle. In Arcturian healing, it is not about imposing energy or intentions of transformation on someone without their consent. Even when the practitioner perceives obvious imbalances in the recipient, it is essential to remember that each being has their own path and rhythm of evolution. For this reason, explicit permission is a requirement before beginning any healing practice. This consent can be given verbally or, in some cases, through a clear energetic intention in situations such as distance healing.

The practitioner must also be aware of the limitations of their role. They are not a savior, nor a master who is above the recipient, but a facilitator who accompanies and supports the healing process. This perspective avoids the creation of unbalanced power dynamics, where the recipient may become dependent on the practitioner. Instead, it fosters the recipient's autonomy, encouraging them to take an active role in their own healing process.

Confidentiality is another essential aspect of ethics in healing. During a session, the recipient may share personal information or experience deep emotions. The practitioner must ensure that this space is safe and that everything that occurs during the session remains in strict confidentiality. This commitment creates an environment of trust where the recipient feels free to open up and participate fully in the process.

The ethical use of Arcturian energies also implies always acting with a pure and selfless intention. Higher energies should not be used for selfish, manipulative purposes or to obtain personal benefits at the expense of others. The Arcturians teach that any attempt to use these energies unethically creates a distortion in the practitioner's energy field, which can generate blockages or imbalances in their own system.

Furthermore, the practitioner should avoid projecting their own expectations or judgments onto the healing process. Each recipient is unique and their healing experience will be different. Some may experience immediate and tangible changes, while others may need time to integrate the energies and notice the effects. The practitioner's role is not to force an outcome, but to trust that the Arcturian energies will work according to what is most appropriate for the recipient at that time.

Self-reflection and self-care are also important components of ethics in healing. Before working with others, the practitioner must ensure that they are in a balanced energetic state and emotionally neutral. If they are dealing with stress, fatigue, or unresolved emotions, these energies can interfere with the practice and negatively impact both the practitioner and the recipient. For this reason, the Arcturians recommend that the practitioner maintain a regular routine of self-healing and energy cleansing practices to stay in an optimal state.

Continuing education is another important aspect of ethics in healing. The practitioner must be committed to their own learning and evolution, constantly seeking to expand their understanding and skills. This includes not only the study of new techniques and concepts, but also the willingness to receive feedback from recipients and reflect on their own practice.

Ethics also extends to interaction with other practitioners and healing systems. The Arcturian holistic system does not seek to compete with other practices, but to complement them and work together for the greater benefit of all. Therefore, it is essential that the practitioner acts with respect towards other traditions and avoids falling into exclusivist or dogmatic attitudes.

Finally, the Arcturians emphasize that healing is an act of unconditional love. This love is not a superficial emotion, but a vibrational force that sustains and nourishes the entire process. The practitioner must cultivate this love in their heart, allowing it to be the guide in all their interactions and decisions.

As the practitioner incorporates these ethical principles into their work, they not only elevate the quality of their healing practices, but also contribute to creating a vibrationally aligned environment with the highest values of the Arcturian system. Ethics is not a series of imposed rules, but a reflection of the pure and conscious intention that drives the healing process, guiding both the practitioner and the recipient to an experience of genuine and lasting transformation.

The human energy body, like the physical body, can accumulate residues that obstruct its optimal functioning. These accumulations can arise from unprocessed emotions, negative mental patterns, interactions with other people, or even from dense environments. Energy cleansing, therefore, is a fundamental practice in the Arcturian holistic healing system, as it ensures that the flow of vital energy is free and harmonious, allowing higher frequencies to work more effectively.

The Arcturians, masters of subtle energy, emphasize that energy cleansing is not an isolated act, but a continuous process that must be integrated into everyday life. Just as the physical body needs regular care to stay healthy, the energy field requires constant attention to ensure its balance and purity.

The first step in energy cleansing is recognizing the need to do so. Signs of a charged or blocked energy field may include unexplained fatigue, irritability, lack of mental clarity, recurring dense emotions, or a general feeling of heaviness. These symptoms should not be ignored, as they act as indicators that the energy system is overloaded and needs to be purified.

One of the simplest and most effective techniques for energy cleansing is guided visualization. In this practice, the practitioner uses their mind to imagine a flow of purifying light passing through their body and energy field, eliminating any stagnant or dense energy. For example, one can visualize a cascade of white light descending from the higher dimensions, washing the body from the crown to the feet and carrying with it any energetic residue to the Earth to be transmuted.

The use of water is another powerful tool in energy cleansing. Water, as a conductor of energy, has the natural ability to absorb and transmute dense energies. A conscious bath, accompanied by the intention to release everything that no longer serves, can be an effective daily practice. As the water flows over the body, the practitioner can visualize it carrying away all accumulated energy charges, leaving them clean and renewed.

Crystals also play an important role in this process. Crystals such as amethyst, clear quartz, and black tourmaline have specific properties that help absorb, transmute, and protect against negative energies. Placing a crystal in the center of the chest while meditating, or even carrying it with you during the day, can act as an energy shield that prevents the accumulation of residues.

Sound, another fundamental vibrational tool, is highly effective for energy cleansing. Instruments such as Tibetan bowls, tuning forks, or bells generate frequencies that resonate with the human energy field, helping to break up blockages and restore harmony. Even a simple clap in the corners of a space can break up stagnant energy and revitalize the environment.

Connection with nature is another powerful method for energy cleansing. Spending time outdoors, especially in contact with elements such as water, earth, or wind, can help release accumulated charges and recharge the energy system with the pure energy of the Earth. Walking barefoot on grass or sand, hugging a tree, or sitting by a river are simple but deeply effective practices to restore balance.

In the context of Arcturian healing, higher frequencies are also a key tool for energy cleansing. These frequencies, channeled from the higher dimensions, act as a solvent that eliminates dense energies and restores the natural flow in the energy system. To work with these frequencies, the practitioner can enter a meditative state and set the intention to receive the purifying energy of the Arcturians, visualizing how these frequencies flow through their body and energy field.

Energy cleansing is not limited to the individual, but can also be applied to physical spaces. The environments in which we live and work accumulate the energy of those who inhabit them and the events that occur in them. A charged house, office, or room can negatively influence the energy state of the people who frequent it. To cleanse a space, tools such as sage, palo santo, or even candles can be used, accompanied by the clear intention to release any unwanted energy.

Another essential aspect of energy cleansing is protection and subsequent maintenance. Once the energy system or a space has been cleansed, it is important to establish an energy shield that prevents the immediate accumulation of new dense energies. This can be achieved by visualizing a protective bubble of light surrounding the body or space, reinforced with the intention of maintaining energy purity.

Consistency is key in these practices. Energy cleansing should not be considered a reactive action in the face of imbalances, but an integral part of personal care. By including these practices in your daily or weekly routine, you create a habit that ensures a strong and balanced energy system, capable of interacting with higher frequencies more fluidly.

Finally, the Arcturians remind us that energy cleansing is a form of spiritual self-care. It not only releases accumulated weight, but also creates an internal space for higher energies to flow and work more effectively. By keeping our energy field clean and balanced, we not only promote our well-being, but also become clearer channels for healing others and connecting with higher dimensions.

Energy cleansing, in its simplicity, is a profoundly transformative practice that strengthens the connection with our purest essence and with the inexhaustible flow of universal energy. With each practice, the energy system is strengthened and aligns more deeply with high vibrations, opening the way for integral and continuous healing.

Chapter 8
Chakras and Self-Healing

Chakras are the energy vortexes that connect the physical body to the energy body, acting as centers of exchange between internal and external vital energy. These essential points not only regulate the energy flow in our system, but also directly influence our physical, emotional, mental, and spiritual health. Chakra harmonization is a fundamental practice within the Arcturian healing system, designed to restore balance and promote alignment with higher frequencies.

Each chakra vibrates at a specific frequency and is associated with a certain color, element, and function. When in balance, the chakras work together as a unified system, allowing energy to flow freely throughout the body. However, factors such as stress, unresolved emotions, trauma, or external imbalances can block or misalign these centers, causing symptoms ranging from physical illness to limiting thought patterns.

The practice of chakra harmonization seeks to restore this balance, helping each energy center vibrate at its optimal frequency. The Arcturians, with their deep knowledge of subtle energy, offer specific frequencies and techniques that can be employed for this purpose, allowing for a profound and lasting transformation in the energy system.

The first step towards harmonization is conscious attunement with the chakras. This begins with the clear intention to balance and revitalize these energy centers. A common practice is to sit in a quiet place, close your eyes, and direct your attention to each chakra, starting from the base of the spine to the top of the head. As you focus your attention on each chakra, you can visualize its associated color, imagining it as a sphere of bright light that rotates evenly.

In the case of the root chakra, for example, one can visualize a vibrant red light at the base of the spine, connecting deeply with the Earth's energy. This center is related to security, stability and connection to the physical plane. By visualizing its light intensifying and rotating smoothly, the practitioner can feel a greater sense of grounding and balance.

The sacral chakra, located just below the navel, is associated with the color orange and regulates emotions, creativity, and interpersonal relationships. Visualizing this center radiating a warm orange light helps release emotional blocks and restore fluidity in these areas.

Each chakra has its own purpose and challenges, and by dedicating time to each one during practice, the practitioner can restore complete energy flow. The combination of visualization, conscious breathing, and intention is one of the most effective tools for this work.

Arcturian frequencies are another essential resource for chakra harmonization. These high vibrations can be channeled directly to the energy centers, promoting their balance and synchronization. To work with these frequencies, the practitioner can enter a meditative state and visualize a ray of light descending from the higher dimensions, touching each chakra and activating it with its purifying energy.

In addition to visualization and frequencies, sound is a powerful tool for harmonization. Each chakra responds to a specific tone, and chanting these tones or listening to recordings that resonate with them can intensify the process. For example, the sound "LAM" is associated with the root chakra, while "OM" is related to the crown chakra. By repeating these sounds while focusing on the corresponding chakras, the practitioner can create a vibrational field that amplifies alignment.

The use of crystals is another common and effective technique. Each crystal has a specific frequency that can resonate with the chakras, helping to balance and energize them. For example, smoky quartz is ideal for working with the root chakra, while amethyst can enhance the crown chakra. Placing these crystals on the chakras during meditation can intensify the connection and accelerate harmonization.

Physical movement can also play an important role in chakra harmonization. Practices such as yoga, tai chi, or even conscious movements designed to activate each energy center can help release blockages and promote the free flow of energy. Gentle movements combined with breath and intention allow the chakras to work in harmony.

In addition to individual techniques, connection with nature is fundamental to this process. Spending time outdoors, feeling the sun, the breeze, or contact with the earth, can restore and revitalize the chakras, especially the lower ones, which are more closely related to the physical plane.

As the practitioner advances in their mastery of chakra harmonization, they may begin to notice subtle but profound changes in their overall well-being. These changes may include greater mental clarity, more balanced emotions, a sense of deeper spiritual connection, and improved physical health. This work not only benefits the practitioner, but also strengthens their ability to work with others as a healing channel.

The Arcturians teach that chakra harmonization is a continuous process. Daily challenges, interactions with others, and external influences can temporarily destabilize the chakras. Therefore, maintaining a regular practice is essential to ensure lasting balance. Even a few minutes a day dedicated to this practice can make a significant difference in the practitioner's quality of life.

Chakra harmonization is not simply a technical exercise, but an act of self-connection and self-love. By dedicating time and energy to this process, the practitioner not only restores balance in their energy system, but also cultivates a deeper relationship with their own essence and with the higher dimensions that support them. It is a transformative practice that opens the door to higher levels of well-being, awareness, and spiritual connection.

Self-healing is the core of any spiritual path, a reminder that the ability to heal resides inherently in every human being. In the Arcturian holistic healing system, this practice not only represents an opportunity to restore inner balance, but also a means to deepen the connection with higher frequencies. The Arcturians, with their infinite wisdom, teach us that healing our own energy system is the first step towards healing the world around us.

Self-healing begins with the conscious intention to create an inner space of harmony and renewal. This act of commitment to oneself establishes the vibrational foundation for higher energies to work effectively. By focusing attention inward, the practitioner not only addresses existing blockages and imbalances, but also strengthens their ability to maintain a balanced energy state amidst everyday challenges.

The first step in the practice of self-healing is to create an environment conducive to energy work. A quiet place, free from distractions and charged with positive intention, can amplify the practitioner's receptivity. Elements such as crystals, candles, high vibration music, or even symbolic images can be used to establish an environment that invites introspection and healing.

A fundamental technique in self-healing is the laying on of hands, an ancestral practice that uses the hands as natural conductors of energy. The practitioner, sitting comfortably, can place their hands on different areas of their body, starting from the head and going down to the feet, while setting the intention to channel purifying and healing energy to each point. During this process, it is important to allow the hands to move intuitively, guided by energetic sensation rather than a rigid pattern.

Conscious breathing is another powerful tool in self-healing. Each inhalation becomes an invitation for higher frequencies to enter the energy system, while each exhalation releases accumulated tension and blockages. A common practice is to visualize a ray of bright light descending from the higher dimensions with each inhalation, filling the body with renewing energy, and with each exhalation, visualize any dense energy leaving the body like gray smoke.

Guided meditation is especially helpful for those beginning their self-healing practice. During these meditations, the practitioner can visualize light of specific colors flowing to different areas of the body, working with the vibration associated with each chakra or energy point. For example, visualizing a green light in the heart area can help release trapped emotions and restore energy flow in this vital center.

The Arcturians teach that self-healing is not limited to the physical body, but also encompasses the energy field. An effective technique for cleansing and strengthening the aura is to visualize a bubble of bright white light surrounding the entire body, acting as a protective shield. As this bubble expands, it takes with it any dense or discordant energy, leaving the energy field clean and vibrant.

Another valuable tool in self-healing is the use of Arcturian symbols. These vibrational patterns, channeled from the higher dimensions, can be drawn on the energy body using the hands or visualized in specific areas that need attention. These symbols act as catalysts that intensify the flow of energy, helping to unblock and realign energy channels.

Sound can also be incorporated into the practice of self-healing. Specific tones, harmonic chants, or even the repetition of mantras vibrate through the energy system, helping to dissolve blockages and raise the overall frequency. Chanting sounds associated with the chakras, such as "OM" for the crown chakra or "RAM" for the solar plexus, can be especially effective in restoring balance.

Connection with nature is another essential aspect of self-healing. Spending time outdoors, feeling the ground beneath your feet, and breathing fresh air allows the energy body to synchronize with the Earth's natural vibrations. This practice, known as grounding, helps release accumulated charges and recharge the energy system with pure, renewing energy.

As the practitioner advances on their self-healing path, it is important to maintain an attitude of patience and self-compassion. Blockages and imbalances may have accumulated over years and do not always release immediately. Each practice, even the briefest, contributes to the overall healing process and strengthens the practitioner's connection to their innate ability to restore balance.

Self-healing also implies a willingness to face and work with the emotions and internal patterns that contribute to imbalances. Instead of avoiding these experiences, the practitioner can use self-healing techniques to explore and transmute these energies, clearing the way for a state of greater harmony.

The Arcturians emphasize that self-healing is not only an act of self-care, but also a means to expand consciousness and raise the overall vibration. As the practitioner strengthens and balances their own energy system, they become a clearer channel for higher frequencies, benefiting not only themselves, but also those around them.

The regular practice of self-healing is an investment in integral well-being and connection with the higher dimensions. By incorporating these techniques into daily life, the practitioner not only promotes their own transformation, but also develops the skills necessary to work with others on the path of healing. Ultimately, self-healing is a reminder that the ability to heal resides within, always accessible to those willing to connect with their essence and with universal energies.

Chapter 9
Sacred Geometry and Channeling

Sacred geometry is the universal language of the cosmos, a manifestation of mathematical and vibrational patterns that underlie all creation. Every shape and structure in the universe, from the spiral of a galaxy to the configuration of a molecule, is influenced by geometric principles that contain a unique and powerful energy. In the Arcturian healing system, sacred geometry acts as a key vibrational tool, allowing energetic alignment, expansion of consciousness, and amplification of healing frequencies.

The Arcturians, masters of the higher dimensions, work with these patterns to channel specific energies to the human system, helping to unblock, balance, and elevate the energy field. Each geometric shape contains an intrinsic meaning and vibrational purpose, functioning as a bridge between the physical and the spiritual. By working with sacred geometry, the practitioner aligns with universal laws, creating a space for deep healing and personal transformation.

One of the most recognized patterns in sacred geometry is the Flower of Life, a symbol composed of intertwined circles that represents the interconnection of all existence. This pattern is an energy map that reflects the underlying structure of the universe. By visualizing or meditating on the Flower of Life, the practitioner can access frequencies that balance the body, mind, and spirit, restoring harmony at all levels of being.

Another key form in sacred geometry is the Merkaba, a three-dimensional symbol that combines two intertwined tetrahedrons, representing the union of masculine and feminine, physical and spiritual. The Merkaba is known for its ability to activate the light body, an advanced energy field that allows connection to higher dimensions. By working with the Merkaba, the practitioner can enhance healing and energy protection, as well as open up to deeper levels of consciousness.

Metatron's Cube is another fundamental pattern that contains all the basic geometric shapes known as the Platonic solids. These forms are associated with the elements of nature and with the structure of physical reality. By working with Metatron's Cube, the practitioner can align their energy with the principles of divine order, promoting stability and clarity in the energy system.

The application of sacred geometry in Arcturian healing includes a variety of practices aimed at amplifying and directing healing energies. One of the most common techniques is geometric visualization, in which the practitioner imagines a specific pattern surrounding their body or an affected area. For example, by visualizing the Flower of Life over the heart, one can balance this energy center and release trapped emotions.

Another powerful practice is the use of physical tools based on sacred geometry, such as crystals carved into specific geometric shapes, pendants, or mandalas. These tools act as vibrational anchors, amplifying intentions and directing energy to specific areas of the body or energy field.

Meditation with sacred geometry is also an effective technique for activating and expanding the energy field. During this practice, the practitioner can focus on a geometric pattern while breathing deeply, allowing their mind to tune into the vibrations inherent in the form. This not only facilitates energy alignment but also raises the overall frequency of the system.

Color, when combined with sacred geometry, further amplifies its effect. Each geometric shape can be visualized in a specific color that resonates with its vibrational purpose. For example, the Merkaba can be visualized in golden light to activate the spiritual connection, while Metatron's Cube in blue can be used to promote calm and clarity.

In the context of Arcturian healing, geometric patterns can be used both in self-healing and in healing others. In a healing session, the practitioner can visualize a geometric pattern over the recipient, channeling Arcturian frequencies through this design. These forms act as energy maps that guide the frequencies to the areas of the system that need them most.

Sacred geometry is not only a healing tool but also a means to expand consciousness. By working with these patterns, the practitioner accesses a deep knowledge about the nature of reality and their own connection to the universe. This understanding not only transforms the energy system but also the perception of oneself and the world, allowing a more complete integration of the higher dimensions into everyday life.

The Arcturians teach us that sacred geometry is a vibrational key that unlocks doors to higher states of being. By integrating these practices into healing, the practitioner not only elevates their own energy system but also becomes a clearer and more effective channel for higher frequencies. Sacred geometry, with its inherent beauty and precision, reminds us that healing is not an isolated event, but a harmonious dance between the human being and the cosmos.

Working with sacred geometry is a transformative experience that opens up new possibilities for healing and spiritual growth. With each practice, the practitioner not only strengthens their connection with Arcturian energies but also deepens their understanding of the universal laws that govern existence. This integration of forms, frequencies, and consciousness guides us to a state of balance, expansion, and fullness that transcends the limits of the physical plane.

Arcturian channeling is a sacred art that allows the practitioner to act as a vibrational bridge between the higher dimensions and the earthly plane. Through this process, the high frequencies and wisdom of the Arcturians flow to the channel, offering guidance, healing, and expansion of consciousness. This act of connection is not a gift reserved for a few, but a latent ability in all human beings, which can be developed through conscious practices and a clear intention.

The essence of channeling lies in the openness and receptivity of the practitioner. The Arcturians, as beings of high vibration, do not interfere with human free will, but expect to be invited with respect and clarity of purpose. The first step to channeling their energies and messages is to establish a sacred space, free from distractions and filled with pure intentions. This space can be physical, such as a quiet place decorated with symbolic elements, or internal, through a state of calm and concentration.

Preparation is key to effective channeling. This includes practices such as meditation, conscious breathing, and connecting with the earth, which help to stabilize the practitioner's energy system and open the subtle channels of perception. A basic technique consists of sitting comfortably, closing your eyes, and visualizing a bright light descending from the cosmos towards the crown of the head, expanding through the body and clearing any blockages or dense energy.

Intention is another essential component of the process. Before beginning, the practitioner should declare their intention to connect with Arcturian energies for the greater good. This intention acts as a vibrational key that aligns the practitioner with the higher frequencies, establishing a safe and clear bridge for channeling.

Once prepared, the practitioner can begin the tuning process. This involves opening oneself to the subtle frequencies and allowing them to flow without resistance. It is common to feel slight vibrations in the body, a feeling of expansion, or even a perception of colors, shapes, or sounds. These experiences vary according to each person's sensitivity, but all indicate that the channel is beginning to align with Arcturian energies.

Channeling can manifest in different ways, depending on the practitioner's skills and preferences. Some experience direct communication in the form of words or ideas that flow through them, while others perceive images, sensations, or energy patterns. In any case, it is important to keep an open mind and not try to control the process, allowing the energies to express themselves naturally.

Automatic writing is a technique commonly used in Arcturian channeling. In this practice, the practitioner holds a pencil or pen over a piece of paper, entering a meditative state while allowing the words to flow without conscious interference. This technique can generate clear and detailed messages, which often contain profound wisdom and practical solutions to specific problems.

Another form of channeling is energy transmission, where the practitioner simply acts as a conduit for Arcturian frequencies. During this process, the energies flow through the practitioner to the recipient, without the need for words or specific actions. This method is especially useful in healing sessions, where Arcturian frequencies work directly on the recipient's energy system to release blockages, balance chakras, and promote overall well-being.

Trust is crucial in channeling. It is common for novice practitioners to question the validity of the perceptions or messages they receive, fearing that they are a product of their imagination. However, the Arcturians teach that trust is built through constant practice and personal validation. Over time, the practitioner will develop a keener sensitivity and inner certainty about the authenticity of the connections.

Ethics also plays a fundamental role in channeling. The practitioner must remember that channeled messages and energies are an act of service, not a tool for control or manipulation. Any information received must be handled with respect and confidentiality, and the recipient's consent must always be obtained before channeling for another person.

The Arcturians remind us that channeling is not limited to specific moments, but that it can be integrated into everyday life. By establishing a constant connection with these higher energies, the practitioner can receive intuitive guidance in daily situations, from personal decisions to interactions with others. This continuous flow of communication not only strengthens the connection with the Arcturians but also raises the practitioner's overall frequency.

As the practitioner advances on their channeling path, they may begin to explore deeper levels of interaction with the Arcturians. This includes working with specific symbols, receiving energy activations, or even collaborating on healing projects for groups or communities. These advanced experiences not only expand the practitioner's skills but also contribute to the balance and evolution of the human collective.

Arcturian channeling is a dynamic and transformative process that connects the practitioner with an inexhaustible source of wisdom, healing, and love. By dedicating time and effort to developing this skill, the practitioner not only expands their own consciousness but also becomes a channel for higher energies that benefit all beings. This act of connection is an expression of the fundamental unity between the individual and the cosmos, reminding us that we are both receivers and transmitters of universal energy.

Through constant practice and pure intention, Arcturian channeling reveals a world of infinite possibilities, where healing, transformation, and enlightenment become accessible to all those willing to open themselves to this experience.

Chapter 10
Auric Healing and Protection

Emotional healing is an essential component of the Arcturian holistic healing system, since emotions are one of the most influential energetic forces in the human body. Often, traumas, painful experiences, and unprocessed emotions become trapped in the energy system, creating blockages that affect emotional, physical, and spiritual well-being. The Arcturians teach that releasing and transmuting these emotional energies is fundamental to restoring balance and advancing on the path of personal evolution.

Emotions are not merely reactions to external stimuli; they are dynamic energies that flow through the body and the energy field. When these energies are expressed and processed in a healthy way, they contribute to a state of balance. However, when they are repressed, ignored, or poorly managed, they can stagnate, generating internal tensions that eventually manifest as illness, stress, or self-limiting behavior patterns.

The first step to emotional healing is the conscious recognition of emotions that are trapped or blocked. This process requires an attitude of self-observation without judgment, allowing emotions to arise and express themselves safely. The Arcturians teach that this acceptance is fundamental, since resisting or denying emotions only strengthens their negative influence on the energy system.

A basic technique for working with emotions is conscious breathing combined with visualization. Upon identifying a blocked emotion, the practitioner can bring their attention to the physical sensation associated with that emotion, such as tightness in the chest or tension in the abdomen. While breathing deeply, they can visualize the energy of the emotion dissolving into a bright light, releasing its charge and allowing it to flow again.

Another powerful tool in emotional healing is introspective writing. The act of writing allows the practitioner to explore their emotions from a place of clarity and detachment. By putting thoughts and feelings on paper, a safe space is created to process and understand them. This practice can also include the ritual burning of the written pages as a symbolic act of release.

Connecting with Arcturian frequencies is especially effective in emotional healing. These high energies work directly with the energy system, dissolving emotional blockages and facilitating their transmutation into higher states of love, compassion, and gratitude. A recommended technique is to sit in meditation, invoke the Arcturian frequencies, and visualize a ray of violet light entering the area of the body where the trapped emotion is perceived. This light acts as a catalyst, cleansing and transforming the energy.

The Arcturians also teach the use of affirmations as emotional reprogramming tools. Statements such as "I accept and release all trapped emotions within me" or "I am at peace with my past and open myself to healing" can be repeated during meditative practices or as part of daily life. These affirmations not only strengthen the practitioner's intention, but also reconfigure emotional vibrations to more harmonious states.

Sound is another vibrational tool that can be used in emotional healing. Specific tones, such as harmonic singing or the sounds of Tibetan bowls, resonate deeply in the energy system, helping to release accumulated emotional tensions. For example, the sound "AH," associated with the heart chakra, can be sung while the practitioner focuses their intention on releasing emotional pain and opening to unconditional love.

Working with the physical body also plays an important role in emotional healing. Unprocessed emotions are often stored in the body as muscle tension or postural patterns. Practices such as yoga, tai chi chuan, or even massage can help release these trapped energies, allowing them to flow again through the system.

Crystals are also valuable allies in emotional healing. Stones such as amethyst, rose quartz, and obsidian have specific properties that can help release, soothe, and transmute dense emotions. Rose quartz, for example, is known for its ability to heal the heart and promote self-love. Placing a crystal on the heart chakra while meditating can intensify emotional release and harmonization.

In the context of emotional healing, the relationship with oneself is fundamental. The Arcturians teach that self-love and self-compassion are essential tools for releasing emotional traumas and preventing new burdens from accumulating. Cultivating a loving relationship with oneself implies practicing forgiveness, both towards others and towards oneself, and recognizing that the path of healing is a continuous process.

In addition to working on a personal level, the Arcturians emphasize the importance of interpersonal relationships in emotional healing. Many trapped emotions have their origin in interactions or bonds with others. Restoring harmony in these relationships, whether through dialogue or through energy release techniques, such as connecting cords, is a crucial part of the process.

Emotional healing is not just a release of past burdens, but also an opening to higher emotional states. As blockages dissolve and dense emotions are transmuted, the practitioner experiences a greater capacity to feel love, gratitude, joy, and compassion. This elevated state not only benefits the individual, but also radiates to their surroundings, contributing to collective well-being.

The Arcturians remind us that emotional healing is an act of courage and love. It requires facing the most vulnerable parts of oneself, but it also offers the reward of deep inner freedom and peace. By releasing trapped emotions and allowing energy to flow, the practitioner not only restores balance in their system, but also creates a space for higher frequencies to work more fully in their life.

Emotional healing, ultimately, is an invitation to return to the core of our essence, where an unconditional love resides that transcends time and wounds. With each practice, the practitioner comes closer to this state of fullness, transforming unresolved emotions into fuel for their spiritual evolution and their connection with the higher dimensions.

The auric field is the first line of energetic defense for the human being, a vibratory emanation that surrounds the physical body and reflects our internal state on multiple levels: physical, emotional, mental, and spiritual. This field not only protects against negative external influences, but also acts as a bridge between the individual and universal energies. In the Arcturian healing system, strengthening and maintaining the auric field is essential to ensure sustained energy balance and a fluid connection with higher frequencies.

The aura is dynamic and continuously responds to our emotions, thoughts, experiences, and the environment. When we are in a state of well-being, the auric field is strong, expansive, and vibrant. However, stress, dense emotions, negative environments, or unhealthy energy connections can weaken it, creating gaps that allow the entry of external influences that destabilize our system.

Strengthening the auric field begins with awareness of its existence and its state. An initial practice consists of sitting in a quiet place and closing your eyes, bringing your attention to the space that surrounds the body. With deep, relaxed breathing, the practitioner can try to perceive their aura, imagining it as a luminous egg that completely surrounds them. Over time, this practice develops a sensitivity that allows you to detect weak areas or inconsistencies in the energy field.

One of the most effective techniques for strengthening the auric field is visualization. The practitioner can imagine themselves surrounded by a bubble of bright white light emanating from their center outward. This bubble acts as a protective shield, repairing any cracks or weaknesses in the aura and ensuring that negative energies cannot penetrate it. This visualization can be repeated daily, especially when starting the day or before entering challenging environments.

Arcturian frequencies also play a fundamental role in strengthening the aura. By channeling these higher energies, the practitioner can cleanse and revitalize their energy field. A recommended practice is to visualize a ray of blue or golden light descending from the higher dimensions and expanding throughout the auric field, filling it with a high and harmonizing vibration.

The use of crystals is another powerful tool for this purpose. Stones such as black tourmaline, amethyst, and clear quartz have specific properties that help protect, cleanse, and amplify the auric field. Placing these crystals in the personal environment, wearing them as jewelry, or using them during meditations can intensify their effect. For example, holding a crystal while visualizing the expansion of the aura can amplify the intention and strengthen the energy shield.

Sound is another effective vibrational technique. Instruments such as Tibetan bowls, tuning forks, or even the human voice generate sound waves that resonate with the auric field, helping to balance and strengthen it. By listening to or producing these sounds, the practitioner can visualize how the vibrations penetrate the aura, dissolving blockages and creating a stable and protective frequency.

Cleansing the aura is also a crucial step in strengthening it. Before reinforcing the energy field, it is important to release any dense or unwanted energy that may be attached to it. Techniques such as using sage or palo santo, bathing with mineral salts, or even the simple act of gently shaking your hands around your body can help cleanse the aura. During this process, intention is fundamental; the practitioner must visualize that any discordant energy dissolves and moves away, leaving the field clean and vibrant.

Connecting with nature is another invaluable practice. Spending time outdoors, especially in natural environments such as forests, rivers, or beaches, recharges the auric field with the pure energy of the Earth. Walking barefoot on the ground, feeling the wind on your skin, or immersing yourself in natural water helps restore energy balance and strengthen the aura naturally.

Caring for the physical body also directly influences the state of the auric field. A balanced diet, regular exercise, and adequate rest are essential to maintain a high vibration at all levels of being. The Arcturians emphasize that the physical body is a reflection of the energy field, and caring for one strengthens the other.

Interpersonal relationships also affect the state of the aura. Being surrounded by people whose vibrations are low or whose intentions are not clear can weaken the energy field. For this reason, it is important to establish healthy boundaries and surround yourself with relationships that nurture and elevate personal energy. When faced with inevitable situations with challenging people or environments, the practitioner can use protection techniques, such as visualizing the bubble of light, to keep their auric field intact.

Strengthening the auric field not only has individual benefits, but also increases the practitioner's ability to interact with higher frequencies. A strong aura acts as a clear channel for Arcturian energies, allowing them to flow freely and work more effectively in healing and spiritual connection.

Furthermore, a strengthened auric field not only protects against negative influences, but also amplifies the practitioner's ability to radiate positive energy to their surroundings. This creates a resonance effect that benefits not only the individual, but also those around them, contributing to collective balance and harmony.

The Arcturians teach that strengthening the auric field is a continuous process, not a single event. By integrating these practices into daily life, the practitioner develops greater energy resilience and a deeper connection with their essence and with the higher dimensions. The aura becomes a vibrant reflection of their inner state and a powerful tool for navigating the world with confidence, clarity, and balance.

As the practitioner strengthens their auric field, they also open themselves to new possibilities for healing and transformation, creating a solid foundation for working with more advanced energies and for expanding their consciousness to higher levels of existence.

Chapter 11
Mental and Energy Healing

The mind, with its ability to shape perceptions, thoughts, and emotions, is one of the most powerful tools of the human being. However, it can also become an obstacle when it gets stuck in negative patterns, limiting beliefs, or reactive habits. In the Arcturian holistic healing system, mental healing focuses on releasing these dysfunctional patterns and cultivating a high mental vibration that promotes well-being, clarity, and connection with higher dimensions.

The first step in mental healing is recognizing that thoughts are not mere internal processes, but expressions of energy that profoundly affect the physical body and the energy system. Negative or repetitive thoughts, such as fear, self-criticism, or doubt, generate density in the energy field, blocking the natural flow of high frequencies. On the other hand, thoughts aligned with love, gratitude, and acceptance amplify the overall vibration, creating an internal space conducive to healing and balance.

Self-observation is a key practice in this process. The Arcturians teach that the first step to healing the mind is to develop awareness of the thoughts that occupy it. This does not mean judging them or resisting them, but simply observing them with curiosity and detachment, as if they were clouds passing through the sky. This act of presence creates a separation between the conscious self and thoughts, allowing the practitioner to choose which to nurture and which to release.

A fundamental technique for mental healing is the reprogramming of negative patterns through positive affirmations. Affirmations, when repeated with intention and conviction, act as vibrational seeds that reconfigure mental energy. For example, phrases such as "I am at peace with myself" or "I choose thoughts that nurture my well-being" can be integrated into daily practices, such as meditation or visualization, to replace dysfunctional mental patterns with ones more aligned with well-being.

Conscious breathing is also a powerful tool for calming the mind and dissolving negative mental patterns. During moments of mental agitation, the practitioner can focus their attention on the breath, inhaling deeply while imagining bright light entering their mind, and exhaling any tension or discordant thoughts. This simple exercise not only relaxes the mind, but also restores energy flow, preparing the practitioner to work with higher frequencies.

The use of Arcturian frequencies is another invaluable resource in mental healing. These energies, vibrating at high levels, have the ability to clear the density accumulated in the mental field and recalibrate its frequency. A recommended practice is to sit in a meditative state, invoke the Arcturian energies, and visualize a ray of golden light descending towards the head, penetrating the mind and dissolving any limiting patterns.

Specific sounds and tones are also effective for working with the mental field. The Arcturians teach that certain frequencies, such as those emitted by Tibetan bowls or bells, resonate directly with the mental system, helping to dissolve density and restore clarity. Listening to these sounds or even singing them can facilitate a vibrational reconfiguration in the mental field.

Another useful technique is introspective writing. Writing thoughts and emotions in a journal allows the practitioner to externalize what occupies their mind, creating space for reflection and release. This process may include exercises such as listing limiting beliefs and then writing opposing affirmations that promote a more positive and expansive mindset.

Physical movement, such as yoga or tai chi chuan, also benefits the mind by releasing accumulated tension in the body that affects the mental state. Gentle movements, combined with conscious breathing, help restore the connection between body and mind, allowing both to work in harmony.

Connection with nature is another essential practice in mental healing. Spending time outdoors, observing natural cycles, and connecting with the elements of the Earth helps to clear the mind and restore its balance. Walking in a forest, feeling the water of a river, or simply observing the sky can provide immediate relief and a broader perspective on mental challenges.

In mental healing, forgiveness is a crucial component. The Arcturians teach that many mental densities stem from unresolved thoughts and emotions in relation to oneself or others. Practicing forgiveness, whether through visualization, affirmations, or symbolic rituals, releases this energetic burden and opens the way to greater clarity and mental peace.

As the practitioner progresses in mental healing, they begin to experience significant changes in their perception and interaction with the world. Thoughts become clearer, emotions stabilize, and a greater ability to focus on the positive and constructive emerges. This elevated state not only benefits the practitioner, but also radiates to their surroundings, creating a resonance effect that raises the collective vibration.

The Arcturians remind us that mental healing is not a destination, but a continuous journey of self-discovery and transformation. With each practice, the practitioner not only releases limiting patterns, but also strengthens their connection with the higher dimensions and with their own divine potential. The mind, when in balance, becomes a powerful ally to manifest a state of harmony and fullness in all aspects of being.

Mental healing is, in essence, an act of empowerment and self-love. By consciously choosing to nurture thoughts that elevate and release those that restrict, the practitioner not only transforms their inner experience, but also opens the door to a fuller life aligned with the higher frequencies of the universe. This process of transformation is an invitation to embrace mental freedom and live from a place of clarity, purpose, and peace.

Energy, in its purest essence, is never static. It flows, transforms, and manifests itself in various ways in the body, mind, and spirit. When this movement is interrupted, energy stagnates, causing imbalances that affect physical, emotional, and spiritual well-being. In the Arcturian healing system, the conscious use of movement and sound is key to unlocking and restoring this natural flow, allowing vital energy to circulate freely and promote integral healing.

Movement, whether physical or vibrational, acts as a catalyst to release energy blocks and reactivate areas of the system that have become inactive. This principle is reflected in ancient and contemporary practices such as yoga, tai chi chuan, and conscious dance, all designed to align the physical body with energy flow. However, the Arcturians offer a unique vibrational approach that combines subtle movements with intention and connection to higher frequencies.

One of the simplest and most effective practices for mobilizing energy is the conscious swaying of the body. The practitioner, standing with feet firmly planted on the ground, can gently sway back and forth or from side to side, feeling how the movement activates the flow of energy from the feet to the top of the head. This movement, accompanied by deep breaths, allows for the release of tension and stimulates the main energy channels.

Spinning is another powerful technique for unlocking and mobilizing energy. Inspired by the circular movements of the dervishes and Arcturian practices, this exercise involves slowly rotating on the axis of the body, with arms outstretched or hands on specific chakras. As the body rotates, the practitioner visualizes energy flowing in a spiral, cleansing and revitalizing the system.

Conscious dance, a freer expression of movement, also has a profound impact on energy. In a safe space, the practitioner can allow the body to move intuitively to the rhythm of music or even in silence, letting the inner energy guide each movement. This act not only releases blockages, but also connects the practitioner with their purest essence, creating a bridge between the physical body and the higher dimensions.

Sound, as a vibrational form of energy, perfectly complements movement in the process of unlocking and healing. Each sound generates a frequency that interacts with the energy field, helping to release densities and restore natural flow. The Arcturians teach that the human voice is one of the most powerful tools for this purpose, since each tone emitted not only affects the practitioner's system, but also the space around them.

A common technique is the chanting of specific tones associated with the chakras. For example, the sound "LAM" resonates with the root chakra, while "OM" is associated with the crown chakra. By chanting these sounds, the practitioner can direct their vibration to specific areas of the body, helping to unblock and revitalize energy flow.

The use of vibrational instruments such as Tibetan bowls, shamanic drums, or bells also amplifies the effect of sound on moving energy. These instruments generate waves that penetrate deeply into the energy system, breaking through blockages and promoting harmonization. For example, playing a drum with a steady rhythm while walking in circles can synchronize the body and energy field, creating a harmonious flow.

Rhythmic breathing is another technique that combines movement and sound to unblock energy. Inspired by Arcturian healing practices, this technique involves inhaling deeply while raising a part of the body, such as the arms, and exhaling while dropping or lowering. This rhythmic movement, accompanied by sounds like a sigh or a chant, stimulates the circulation of vital energy throughout the system.

The Arcturians also emphasize the importance of working with the environment to amplify the movement of energy. Open spaces, such as a field or a beach, allow the body and energy field to expand without restriction. In these environments, the practitioner can walk barefoot, move their arms in wide circles, or even jump gently, feeling the energy flow through them and towards the Earth.

Water is an element that naturally promotes energy movement. The Arcturians recommend practices such as walking in a shallow river, moving gently in a pool, or even simply letting the body float in the water. This contact with water stimulates energy flow while cleansing and renewing the system.

The role of intention is fundamental in all these practices. Both movement and sound become more effective when the practitioner sets a clear intention, such as releasing blockages, strengthening energy flow, or aligning with higher frequencies. Intention acts as a vibrational guide that directs energy towards the desired purpose, amplifying the impact of the techniques.

As the practitioner integrates movement and sound into their daily life, they begin to experience greater fluidity and lightness in their energy system. Blockages that once seemed insurmountable dissolve, and the body, mind, and spirit feel more aligned and connected. This fluidity not only benefits the individual, but also enhances their ability to work with others and effectively channel higher energies.

The Arcturians teach us that energy in motion is the essence of life. By unblocking energy flow, the practitioner not only restores their inner balance, but also attunes to the natural rhythm of the universe, opening a path to greater harmony, expansion, and fulfillment. These practices, while simple in appearance, have the power to profoundly transform the practitioner, reminding them that true healing comes from within, through the constant and free flow of vital energy.

Chapter 12
Remote Healing and Sacred Spaces

Remote healing is a clear manifestation of the universal principle that energy is not limited by time or space. In the Arcturian holistic healing system, this practice allows high frequencies to be channeled to other people, regardless of their physical location, creating a vibrational bridge that facilitates healing and balance. This method, deeply respected and used by the Arcturians, expands the possibilities of healing, bringing support and harmonization to those who cannot be physically present.

The foundation of remote healing lies in the understanding that everything in the universe is interconnected through a unified energy field. This field, known in various traditions as the cosmic web or the universal matrix, allows energy to flow between beings without restrictions of space. The Arcturians teach that by establishing a clear and focused intention, the practitioner can access this field and direct the frequencies to the recipient with precision and effectiveness.

The first step in the practice of remote healing is the preparation of the practitioner's energy space. This space should be quiet, free from distractions, and charged with a clear and positive intention. Elements such as crystals, candles, soft music or sacred symbols can help raise the vibration of the environment, creating a conducive place for channeling higher energies.

Connecting to the earth is essential before starting any remote healing practice. The practitioner can visualize energy roots extending from their feet to the Earth's core, ensuring a balanced and stable flow of energy. This anchoring not only protects the practitioner from possible energy overloads, but also reinforces their ability to act as a clear and effective channel.

Once the space is prepared, the practitioner sets the intention to connect with the recipient. This intention can be expressed silently or aloud, formulating a statement such as: "I connect with [recipient's name] to channel healing energy in alignment with their highest good." This statement creates a vibrational bridge that links the practitioner with the recipient's energy field.

Visualization is a powerful tool in remote healing. The practitioner can imagine the recipient as if they were in front of them, surrounded by a bright light that represents their energy field. While channeling Arcturian frequencies, one can visualize these energies flowing from their hands or heart to the recipient, filling them with light and restoring balance in all areas of their being.

The use of sacred symbols can also enhance the effectiveness of remote healing. The Arcturians teach that certain geometric patterns and symbols act as energy portals that intensify the flow of energy.

Drawing or visualizing these symbols in the recipient's energy space can help direct and focus frequencies to specific areas that need attention.

During practice, the practitioner may feel subtle sensations that indicate energy exchange, such as warmth in the hands, gentle vibrations, or intuitive images related to the recipient. These perceptions are not mandatory, but they act as signs that the connection is active and that the energies are flowing.

The time spent on remote healing varies according to the needs of the recipient and the intuition of the practitioner. However, 10 to 20 minutes is usually sufficient for an effective session. Upon completion, it is important to consciously close the energy connection. This can be done by thanking the recipient and the universe for the opportunity to channel the energies and visualizing the vibrational bridge gently dissolving.

Energy protection is crucial after each session. The practitioner can visualize a protective bubble of light surrounding them, ensuring that any unwanted residual energy is transmuted or released. It is also advisable to perform an energy cleansing, such as shaking the hands or washing the palms with cold water, to restore neutrality to the practitioner's energy field.

It is important to remember that remote healing should always be performed with the recipient's consent. Although the intention behind the practice is positive, respecting the recipient's free will is a fundamental ethical principle in the Arcturian system. In cases where it is not possible to obtain explicit consent, such as with unconscious people or in emergency situations, one can set the intention that the energies will only be used if the recipient is willing to receive them.

Remote healing benefits not only the recipient, but also the practitioner, strengthening their ability to work with higher energies and deepening their connection to the unified field. In addition, this practice allows Arcturian frequencies to reach places and people who would not otherwise be able to access them, expanding their transformative impact on the world.

The Arcturians teach us that remote healing is a reminder of our universal interconnectedness. Through this practice, the practitioner becomes a conscious channel of love and balance, bringing light to those who need it most, regardless of physical barriers. This act not only transforms the recipient, but also raises the collective vibration, contributing to planetary well-being and harmony.

With each session, remote healing reinforces the fundamental truth that energy transcends all boundaries and that, by aligning ourselves with higher frequencies, we can touch lives, heal hearts and transform realities, even from a distance.

The spaces we inhabit are extensions of our energy field, reflections of our emotions, thoughts and experiences. An environment charged with unbalanced energies can affect our physical, emotional and spiritual health, limiting our ability to connect with higher dimensions. In the Arcturian holistic healing system, environmental healing is an essential practice that not only cleanses and harmonizes physical spaces, but also establishes a high energy flow that sustains those who inhabit them.

Every space has an inherent vibration that is influenced by several factors: the people who occupy it, the emotions generated within it, the objects present and even the events that took place there. Dense energies, such as stress, anger or pain, can accumulate in an environment, creating blockages that affect the quality of life and hinder the flow of higher frequencies. Environmental healing seeks to release these densities, restoring harmony and raising the vibration of the space.

The first step to healing an environment is to recognize its energy state. This can be done through conscious observation, paying attention to how the space feels. Are there areas that seem heavier or uncomfortable? Is it possible to perceive emotions or memories associated with certain places? The Arcturians teach that developing this sensitivity to the environment is key to identifying areas that need attention.

One of the most common tools for energetic cleansing of spaces is the use of sacred smoke, such as that of white sage or palo santo. These plants have vibrational properties that dissolve and transmute dense energies, leaving the environment clean and revitalized. During this practice, the practitioner can walk through the space holding the lit plant, allowing the smoke to flow to the corners, doors and windows, while establishing a clear intention of release and harmonization.

Sound is another powerful tool for environmental healing. Vibrational instruments, such as Tibetan bowls, shamanic drums or bells, generate frequencies that penetrate deeply into the energy field of space, breaking up blockages and promoting a balanced flow. By playing these instruments in different areas of the environment, the practitioner can amplify their effect by combining them with the intention of raising the vibration of the place.

Light, both natural and symbolic, is fundamental to the healing of spaces. Opening the windows to allow sunlight to enter not only purifies the environment, but also fills it with vital energy. On a symbolic level, lighting candles or visualizing rays of golden light flowing into the space acts as a catalyst for the transmutation of dense energies.

Physical cleansing also directly influences the energy state of an environment. Clutter and accumulated objects can retain and stagnate energy, preventing its natural flow. The Arcturians recommend a deep and conscious cleaning, during which the practitioner can set the intention to release not only unnecessary physical objects, but also the energies they may have accumulated.

Crystals are valuable allies in environmental healing. Stones such as amethyst, clear quartz and black tourmaline can be strategically placed in space to absorb, transmute and stabilize energies. For example, placing a clear quartz in the center of a room can act as an amplifier of high vibrations, while a black tourmaline near the door protects the space from negative external influences.

Sacred geometry is another vibrational tool that can be used to harmonize spaces. Geometric patterns, such as the Flower of Life or the Metatron's Cube, can be physically represented in the environment, whether as decorations, mandalas or even traced in the air through visualization. These patterns act as energy portals that connect the space with higher dimensions, stabilizing and raising its vibration.

The use of water is also effective in cleaning and revitalizing an environment. A container with salt water can be placed in a corner or in the center of the room for a certain time, allowing it to absorb dense energies. Afterwards, the water should be discarded respectfully, preferably in a place where it can be transmuted, such as the earth.

Intention and connection with Arcturian frequencies are at the core of any environmental healing practice. Before beginning, the practitioner can invoke these higher energies, visualizing a ray of blue or golden light descending from the higher dimensions into space, cleansing it and filling it with high vibrations. This intention establishes a vibrational bridge that allows Arcturian frequencies to work directly in the environment.

Environmental healing not only restores harmony, but also creates a space that supports the well-being and spiritual expansion of those who inhabit it. An energetically balanced environment acts as a vibrational refuge, facilitating connection with higher dimensions and strengthening the individual energy system.

In addition, the Arcturians teach that the healing of spaces has a collective impact, since each harmonized environment contributes to the overall balance of the planet. By cleansing and raising the vibration of the spaces we inhabit, we not only benefit individually, but also contribute to a more balanced and positive energy flow in the world.

The constant practice of environmental healing is an act of care and respect for ourselves and for the space we share with others. With each cleansing and harmonization, the practitioner not only transforms the environment, but also strengthens their connection with higher frequencies, remembering that true healing is an act of collaboration between the individual, their environment and the universe.

Chapter 13
Multidimensional Healing and Energy Fusion

As the practitioner delves deeper into the Arcturian healing system, new possibilities open up for working with more complex and multidimensional energies. Advanced practices are the next step on this path, offering tools and techniques that allow one to explore higher levels of healing, connection, and transformation. These practices require a solid foundation in the fundamentals already covered, as well as a constant commitment to ethics, intention, and spiritual preparation.

One of the pillars of advanced practices is multidimensional healing. The Arcturians teach that energy imbalances do not always originate on the physical or emotional plane, but can have roots in other dimensions of being, such as the mental, spiritual, or even in past or future timelines. Multidimensional healing involves accessing these levels and working directly on them to release blockages and restore harmony.

To begin with this practice, the practitioner must enter a state of deep meditation, using previously learned connection techniques. During this meditation, one can visualize ascending a ladder of light or moving through a portal to a higher dimension. In this elevated energetic space, the practitioner sets the intention to identify and heal any imbalances that may be affecting the recipient, whether it be themselves or another person.

Working with timelines is an extension of multidimensional healing. Blockages or dysfunctional patterns that manifest in the present often have their origin in past events or future projections. By connecting with Arcturian frequencies, the practitioner can access these timelines, identifying the key points that need healing and directing energy to them. This work does not alter the events that occurred, but transforms their energetic impact, freeing the recipient from emotional or karmic burdens.

Integrating specific frequencies is another advanced practice in the Arcturian system. Each vibrational frequency has a unique purpose, such as cleansing, protecting, activating, or transforming. The Arcturians transmit these frequencies through specific visualizations, sounds, or symbols that the practitioner can use in their sessions. For example, the violet frequency is ideal for transmuting dense energies, while the golden frequency promotes connection with universal wisdom.

The use of complex geometric patterns, such as dynamic mandalas or three-dimensional structures, is also a feature of advanced practices. These patterns act as energy maps that guide the flow of frequencies to specific areas of the energy system. In a session, the practitioner can visualize a geometric pattern floating above the recipient, rotating and adjusting to activate energy centers or unblock channels.

Another advanced tool is the activation of the light body. This energy body, also known as the Merkaba in some traditions, is a vibrational structure that connects the individual with the higher dimensions and with their divine essence. Activating the light body allows the practitioner not only to access higher levels of consciousness, but also to channel higher energies more effectively.

To activate the light body, the practitioner can visualize two intertwined tetrahedrons, one pointing up and the other down, rotating around them. During this visualization, the intention is set to activate this structure, allowing Arcturian frequencies to flow through it. This process not only raises the overall vibration of the practitioner, but also strengthens their energy field and protects them from negative external influences.

Working with groups is another aspect of advanced practices. When several people come together with a common intention of healing, the collective energy field amplifies the impact of the channeled frequencies. In these sessions, the practitioner can act as a facilitator, guiding the group through meditations, visualizations, and channeling that benefit both individuals and the collective.

The Arcturians also teach that advanced practices include conscious collaboration with guides and spiritual masters. These high vibrational beings offer guidance, protection, and energetic support during sessions. Establishing a connection with these guides requires a clear intention and a willingness to listen and follow their wisdom. During a session, the practitioner can invoke the Arcturian masters, asking them to work directly with the recipient to address imbalances at a deeper level.

Finally, integration is a crucial component of advanced practices. As the practitioner works with higher energies and more complex techniques, it is essential to take time to assimilate and balance the experiences. This includes grounding practices, adequate rest, and self-reflection to ensure that the integrated energies flow harmoniously within the practitioner's energy system.

Advanced practices are not an end in themselves, but a means to deepen the path of healing and spiritual connection. The Arcturians remind us that true mastery lies not in the complexity of the techniques, but in the pure intention and ethical commitment to the well-being of all beings. As the practitioner incorporates these tools and techniques into their work, they not only expand their skills and understanding, but also become a clearer and more powerful channel for higher frequencies. This journey towards the advanced is an invitation to explore the vast possibilities of the energetic universe, always guided by love, compassion, and the purpose of serving the greater good.

Energy fusion is an advanced approach in the Arcturian healing system, in which different techniques, frequencies, and methods are integrated to create a synergistic flow of energy. This practice allows the practitioner to combine elements of various healing systems, such as laying on of hands, visualization, sound and sacred geometry, with Arcturian frequencies. The result is a unique healing experience that amplifies the effectiveness of the tools used, adapting to the specific needs of the recipient or the environment.

The fundamental principle behind energy fusion is interconnection. The Arcturians teach that all forms of energy are intertwined and that the most effective healing occurs when these energies work together harmoniously. Energy fusion, therefore, is not about randomly overlapping techniques, but about recognizing how each element contributes to overall balance and consciously using it in synergy with others.

Preparation for energy fusion begins with the clear intention of the practitioner. Before a session, the practitioner can reflect on the specific needs of the recipient or space, identifying the areas that require attention and choosing the techniques that best suit them. This process may include creating a flexible plan that allows for intuitive adjustments during the session.

One of the key aspects of energy fusion is the combination of frequencies. Each technique or vibrational tool has its own inherent frequency, and the practitioner must learn to work with these vibrations consciously. For example, while using crystals like rose quartz to work with the heart chakra, the practitioner can simultaneously channel Arcturian frequencies aimed at releasing trapped emotions, maximizing the impact on this energy center.

Sound is a tool that lends itself naturally to energy fusion. By using instruments such as Tibetan bowls, drums or bells, the practitioner can combine sound vibrations with Arcturian visualizations or symbols, intensifying the energy flow. For example, during a session, the practitioner could play a Tibetan bowl while visualizing a specific geometric pattern floating above the recipient, amplifying the resonance in their energy system.

Sacred geometry also plays an important role in energy fusion. Geometric patterns act as vibrational maps that guide the flow of energy to specific areas of the recipient's system. During a session, the practitioner can integrate the visualization of a mandala with the use of physical tools, such as crystals placed at strategic points around the recipient. This combination allows energies to work together coherently to restore balance.

Conscious physical movement is another element that can be integrated into energy fusion. Practices such as yoga, tai chi chuan or even intuitive movements can be used to unblock and mobilize energy in the body, while the practitioner channels Arcturian frequencies to the recipient. This approach not only benefits the recipient, but also helps the practitioner to maintain their own balanced energy during the session.

Energy fusion also includes the integration of techniques from different healing traditions. The Arcturians teach that all spiritual and energy practices, when used with pure intention, are expressions of the same universal flow. Therefore, the practitioner can incorporate elements from traditions such as Reiki, shamanic healing or sound therapy, combining them with Arcturian frequencies to create a unique and holistic approach.

A practical example of this integration would be to combine the laying on of hands with the use of mantras or sacred chants. While the practitioner places their hands on the recipient, they can sing or recite a specific mantra that resonates with the energy center in question. At the same time, they can visualize a beam of golden light flowing through their hands to the recipient, uniting the power of sound, intention and channeled energy into a single coherent flow.

Intuition is fundamental in energy fusion. While technical knowledge and preparation are important, the practitioner must be open to intuitive adjustments during the session. The Arcturians emphasize that energy works most effectively when it flows freely, without restrictions imposed by rigid expectations. Listening to the recipient's signals and allowing the energies to guide themselves is an essential aspect of this practice.

Closure and integration are crucial steps in energy fusion. Once multiple techniques and frequencies have been worked with, the practitioner must ensure that the energies are balanced and fully integrated into the recipient's system. This can be achieved by visualizing a soft light that envelops the recipient's entire body, stabilizing the energy flow and ensuring that the effects of the session are long-lasting.

In addition, the Arcturians remind us that energy fusion not only benefits the recipient, but also the practitioner. By combining techniques and working with high frequencies, the practitioner deepens their connection to higher energies and strengthens their own energy field. This process is an ongoing learning experience, where each session brings new insights and skills.

Energy fusion is a creative and transformative act that allows the practitioner to explore the infinite possibilities of working with energy. By integrating techniques, frequencies and tools with intention and awareness, a unique vibrational flow is created that not only heals, but also raises the vibration of all involved. This practice, in essence, is a celebration of the unity and interconnection of all forms of energy, reminding us that healing is an ever-evolving art.

Chapter 14
Collective Healing and Intuition

Collective healing represents a powerful act of energetic collaboration, in which the intentions, vibrations, and frequencies of multiple individuals converge to generate a transformative impact on groups, communities, and even the planetary energy field. In the Arcturian holistic healing system, this practice not only elevates the vibration of the participants but also acts as a catalyst for balance and harmonization on a larger scale.

The Arcturians teach that the collective energy field amplifies individual energies, creating a stronger and more effective vibrational flow. When a group comes together with a common intention of healing, the generated frequencies transcend individual boundaries and penetrate the deepest layers of the group energy field, dissolving blockages and promoting a state of harmony.

The first step in collective healing is to establish a clear and shared purpose. This purpose can range from healing a specific group to providing energetic support to a region in crisis or raising the planetary vibration. Clarity of intention acts as a vibrational guide that aligns the energies of all participants, creating a coherent and powerful flow.

Preparation is essential for a collective healing session. This includes both the physical space and the energetic state of the participants. The location where the session takes place should be quiet, clean, and conducive to concentration. Elements such as candles, crystals, sacred symbols, or high-frequency music can help raise the vibration of the space.

Each participant should prepare their own energy system before the session. This includes grounding practices, conscious breathing, and intention alignment. The Arcturians recommend that participants engage in a brief group meditation at the beginning, visualizing a ray of light descending from the higher dimensions towards the group, connecting everyone present in a unified energy field.

Visualization is a central tool in collective healing. During the session, participants can unite in a guided visualization that represents the shared purpose. For example, if the goal is to send healing energy to an affected community, the group can imagine a golden ray of light flowing from the center of the group towards the specific region, enveloping it in love, peace, and balance.

The use of sound and vibration significantly amplifies the impact of collective healing. Instruments such as Tibetan bowls, shamanic drums, or tuning forks can be played in synchrony with the group's intentions, generating a resonance that penetrates deeply into the collective energy field. Additionally, participants can chant mantras or specific tones that align with the purpose of the session, strengthening the vibrational flow.

Sacred geometry is another powerful tool in collective healing. Geometric patterns, such as the Flower of Life or the Merkaba, can be visualized or physically represented in the group space. These patterns act as vibrational portals that channel higher frequencies into the collective field, intensifying the impact of the session.

During the practice, intuition plays a crucial role. While certain structures or techniques can be planned, it is important that the group remains open to spontaneous adjustments guided by the energies present. The Arcturians teach that higher frequencies often guide the flow of the session, showing specific areas that need attention or revealing patterns that need to be released.

Completion and closure are critical steps in collective healing. At the conclusion of the session, it is essential that the group takes time to stabilize and seal the generated energies. This can be done through a group visualization in which everyone imagines a field of light surrounding and protecting the purpose that was worked on. Furthermore, expressing gratitude to the higher energies and the participants for their contribution strengthens the impact of the practice.

The effects of collective healing are not limited to the group or the immediate recipient. The Arcturians explain that the frequencies generated in these sessions expand beyond time and space, influencing the balance of the planetary energy field. Each act of collective healing contributes to global well-being, acting as a vibrational beacon that raises consciousness and promotes universal harmony.

Furthermore, collective healing sessions have a transformative effect on the participants. By contributing to the well-being of the group or a greater cause, individuals strengthen their own connection to the higher frequencies, experience an expansion of their energy field, and develop a deeper sense of unity with others and the universe.

The Arcturians remind us that collective healing does not require a specific number of participants or advanced technical complexity. Even a small group with a clear intention can generate a significant impact. The most important thing is the purity of intention and the commitment of the participants to the shared purpose.

Ultimately, collective healing is an expression of universal interconnectedness. Through this practice, the group not only transforms the energy field around it but also becomes a channel for the higher frequencies that benefit all of creation. This act of energetic collaboration is a reminder that true healing occurs when we work together, guided by love and the desire to contribute to the greater good.

Intuition is one of the most valuable tools in the Arcturian healing system, a bridge between the conscious mind and the higher dimensions. Developing this innate gift allows the practitioner to tune into subtle energies, receive clear messages, and act with precision during healing practices. The Arcturians teach that intuition is not a privilege of a few, but an inherent ability of all human beings, which can be cultivated through practice, openness, and conscious intention.

Intuitive development begins with the recognition that intuition is not limited to a specific channel, such as vision or inner hearing. Each individual has their own intuitive style, which can manifest as bodily sensations, mental images, inner words, or simply an inexplicable certainty. Understanding and accepting these differences is key to strengthening this connection.

The first step to developing intuition is to create an inner space of calm and receptivity. A noisy mind and stress block intuitive messages, so practices such as meditation and conscious breathing are fundamental. During these practices, the practitioner can focus on inner silence, allowing thoughts to dissolve and creating a clear channel to receive intuitive impressions.

A basic technique to stimulate intuition is the practice of inner questioning. The practitioner can formulate a clear and specific question, such as "What do I need to know about this situation?" or "What is the next step on my path?". Then, enter a state of calm, paying attention to the first impressions that arise, whether they are images, words, sensations, or emotions. It is important not to analyze or judge these answers, but simply receive them as they come.

The Arcturians teach that intuition is strengthened with the constant practice of conscious observation. This implies paying attention to the small details of daily life, such as repetitive patterns, coincidences, or inner sensations in the face of certain people or situations. This exercise not only improves intuitive perception but also trains the practitioner to trust their subtle impressions.

Connection with Arcturian frequencies is a powerful catalyst for intuitive development. During a meditation, the practitioner can visualize a ray of blue light descending from the higher dimensions towards their crown, opening and activating the intuitive channels. This practice not only clears energetic blockages but also attunes the practitioner to the higher vibrations, facilitating the reception of clear messages.

The use of vibrational tools, such as crystals or sacred symbols, can also support intuitive development. Crystals such as amethyst, labradorite, or clear quartz have specific properties that amplify intuitive abilities. Placing a crystal on the third eye during meditation or carrying it as an amulet can intensify the connection to higher energies.

Intuitive journaling is another effective tool for strengthening this ability. By regularly writing about thoughts, impressions, and perceived messages, the practitioner not only trains their intuition but also develops a valuable record of patterns and synchronicities that can guide their path. This habit reinforces trust in inner perceptions and facilitates the integration of intuition into daily life.

The body is an important ally in intuitive development. Physical sensations, such as tightness in the chest, tingling in the abdomen, or warmth in the hands, often act as intuitive signals. Learning to listen to and understand these bodily responses is essential to interpreting energetic messages effectively.

Another advanced technique to enhance intuition is the practice of directed visualization. During meditation, the practitioner can imagine a symbolic landscape, such as a garden or a temple, and explore this inner space in search of messages. The objects, colors, or figures that appear in these visualizations often contain relevant information for the practitioner's current situation.

Intuitive development is not just about receiving information, but also about acting on it with confidence. The Arcturians teach that every time the practitioner follows their intuition, they strengthen the connection with this ability and send a clear message to the universe that they are ready to receive more guidance. Even small steps and seemingly insignificant decisions can strengthen this vibrational bond.

Connection with nature is another key practice for intuitive development. Spending time outdoors, observing the flow of natural life, helps to tune into the universal rhythm and release mental blocks. The Arcturians recommend simple practices such as walking barefoot on the earth, observing the night sky, or listening to the sounds of a river as ways to open intuitive channels.

Intuitive development is a continuous process that requires patience, dedication, and self-compassion. It is not about achieving an ideal state, but about exploring and strengthening this connection over time. Mistakes or misinterpretations are a natural part of the path, and each experience, regardless of the outcome, contributes to the practitioner's growth.

The Arcturians remind us that intuition is not just a tool for healing or decision-making, but also a gateway to a deeper connection with the higher self and the higher dimensions. As the practitioner strengthens this ability, they experience greater clarity, confidence, and fluidity on their path, opening up new possibilities for growth and spiritual expansion.

Intuition, in its essence, is a reminder that the answers and guidance are always available within us. By developing this gift, the practitioner not only transforms their own experience but also becomes a clearer and more effective channel for the higher frequencies, bringing light and clarity to the world around them.

Chapter 15
Crystals and Arcturian Healing

Crystals have been recognized throughout history as sacred tools, carriers of energies that interact with the human energy field and the frequencies of the universe. In the Arcturian holistic healing system, crystals are not just physical objects, but also vibrational manifestations that act as bridges between dimensions. Their ability to amplify, store, and direct energy makes them indispensable allies for enhancing healing practices and elevating the connection to higher frequencies.

Each crystal has a unique composition and an inherent geometric structure that defines its vibration. The Arcturians teach that this vibration interacts with the human energy field, harmonizing, cleansing, and strengthening the flow of energy. In addition, crystals can be programmed with specific intentions, which makes them versatile and customizable tools in healing practices.

The first step in working with crystals is to select those that resonate with the desired purpose. For example, clear quartz is known for its ability to amplify energy and intention, while amethyst promotes calm, mental clarity, and spiritual connection. Rose quartz, on the other hand, works with the heart chakra, facilitating emotional healing and self-love. The Arcturians recommend choosing crystals not only for their known function, but also by trusting intuition, allowing the practitioner to be guided to the crystal they need at that moment.

Before using a crystal, it is essential to cleanse it energetically to release any residual vibration it may have absorbed. There are several techniques for this, such as passing the crystal through the smoke of sage or palo santo, briefly submerging it in salt water (if its composition allows), or exposing it to sunlight or moonlight. During this process, the practitioner should set the intention to purify the crystal, visualizing how the dense energy dissolves and is transmuted.

Programming crystals is a key practice in the Arcturian system. This involves establishing a clear intention and charging the crystal with that intention so that it acts as a specific vibrational channel. To do this, the practitioner can hold the crystal in their hands, closing their eyes and visualizing the intention entering its structure, as if light were impregnating each facet of the mineral. For example, a clear quartz can be programmed to amplify energy during a healing session, or a black obsidian to protect against negative external influences.

Crystals can be placed directly on the body during a healing session, aligning them with the chakras or specific areas that need attention. For example, placing an amethyst on the third eye can help calm the mind and facilitate intuitive opening, while a black tourmaline on the root chakra strengthens the connection to the earth and protects the energy field.

In working with crystals, sacred geometry amplifies their effects. By arranging the crystals in geometric patterns, such as the Flower of Life or the Merkaba, an energy field is created that enhances harmonization and connection with higher frequencies. These arrangements can be made around the recipient, on an altar, or even as a visualization during meditation.

The use of crystals in combination with other vibrational tools, such as sound or Arcturian frequencies, is another advanced technique in this work. For example, during a healing session, the practitioner can play a Tibetan singing bowl while directing energy to a programmed crystal, allowing the vibrations of the sound and the crystal to combine to amplify the energetic impact.

Crystals are also useful in healing environments. Placing them strategically in different areas of a space can balance and raise the overall vibration. For example, a rose quartz in the bedroom promotes calm and love, while an amethyst near a window can transmute dense external energies before they enter the home.

Working with crystals is not limited to formal healing sessions. Practitioners can carry crystals with them during the day, as amulets or in pockets, to maintain a high vibration and protect their energy field. The Arcturians teach that crystals act as energetic companions, reminding us of our connection to the Earth and to the higher dimensions.

As the practitioner deepens their relationship with crystals, they may experience more intuitive communication with them. Each crystal has a unique energetic "personality", and by working with them regularly, the practitioner can begin to perceive impressions, messages, or sensations that guide their use. This interaction strengthens the vibrational connection and allows for more precise and effective work.

Care and respect for crystals are fundamental on this path. The Arcturians emphasize that these minerals are not mere objects, but vibrational companions that respond to the energy and intention of the practitioner. Keeping them clean, charged, and in a special place ensures that they remain vibrationally active and ready for use.

Crystals, in essence, are tangible reminders of the connection between the physical and the energetic. By working with them, the practitioner not only amplifies their ability to channel and direct energy, but also deepens their understanding of the vibrational interactions that sustain the universe. In the Arcturian system, crystals are much more than tools; they are allies that connect us with the wisdom of the Earth and with the higher dimensions, helping us to heal, transform, and raise our vibration to states of greater harmony and fullness.

Anchoring light is a central practice in the Arcturian holistic healing system, designed to establish a stable and continuous flow of higher energies in the practitioner's energy system and surroundings. This process involves channeling high frequencies from the higher dimensions to the physical plane, creating a vibrational bridge that not only restores balance and harmony, but also acts as a beacon of light for those around you.

The Arcturians teach that anchoring light is not a passive act, but an active collaboration between the practitioner and universal forces. Through this practice, the practitioner becomes a conscious channel for higher energies, helping to integrate these frequencies into their body, mind and spirit, as well as into the environment where they are.

The first step to anchoring light is to prepare the inner and outer space. This begins with a personal energy cleansing, using techniques such as conscious breathing, visualization of purifying light, or the use of specific crystals such as clear quartz or amethyst. At the same time, it is important to cleanse and harmonize the physical environment, ensuring that the space is free of distractions and dense energies.

Once the space is prepared, the practitioner sets a clear intention for anchoring light. This intention acts as a vibrational guide that aligns the practitioner with the higher frequencies. It can be formulated in words, such as "I open myself to channel and anchor light for the highest good of all beings", or simply held as a clear and sincere inner intention.

Visualization is a key tool in this process. During practice, the practitioner can imagine a ray of bright light descending from the higher dimensions to their crown, flowing through their body and extending towards the Earth. This visualization not only strengthens the connection with higher energies, but also helps to integrate these frequencies into the practitioner's energy system.

The use of Arcturian symbols can amplify the impact of anchoring light. These symbols, which act as vibrational portals, can be visualized floating above the practitioner or drawn with the hands in the energy space. Each symbol has a specific frequency that guides and structures the flow of light, ensuring that it integrates in a balanced and harmonious way.

Conscious breathing is another powerful tool during light anchoring. By inhaling deeply, the practitioner can imagine that the light enters their body, filling every cell and every energy space. Upon exhaling, they visualize that this light expands into their surroundings, radiating love, peace and balance. This breathing cycle helps to establish a constant flow of energy that connects the practitioner with the higher dimensions and with the Earth.

Anchoring light not only benefits the practitioner, but also the environment in which it is performed. The Arcturians teach that this practice has an impact on the energy field of the space, raising its vibration and creating an environment conducive to healing, meditation and spiritual growth. For this reason, it is recommended to practice anchoring light regularly in homes, workplaces or any space where dense energies or imbalances are perceived.

Furthermore, light anchoring can be used as a healing tool for others. During a session, the practitioner can visualize that the light flows to the recipient, filling their energy field with high frequencies. This act not only promotes healing and balance in the recipient, but also strengthens their connection with higher energies.

Conscious physical movement can be integrated into the practice of anchoring light to intensify its effect. For example, raising your arms towards the sky while inhaling, and lowering them towards the Earth while exhaling, reinforces the visualization of the flow of light and helps to integrate the frequencies into the physical body.

Consistency is essential in anchoring light. Although a single practice can generate a significant impact, the Arcturians teach that regular repetition of this practice strengthens the connection with higher energies and establishes a stable and lasting flow. Even a few minutes a day dedicated to anchoring light can profoundly transform the practitioner's energy system and their surroundings.

Anchoring light can also be done in collective situations, such as group meetings or healing events. In these cases, the combined energy of the participants amplifies the impact of the practice, creating a collective vibrational field that benefits not only those present, but also the environment and the planetary energy grid.

The effects of anchoring light are not always immediate or visible, but the Arcturians assure that each practice contributes to the balance and evolution of the global energy field. This act of service not only transforms the practitioner, but also radiates to the world, acting as a tangible reminder of universal interconnectedness.

Anchoring light is, in essence, an act of loving collaboration between the practitioner and universal forces. By practicing it, the practitioner not only raises their own vibration, but also becomes a channel for higher frequencies, bringing light and harmony to all levels of existence. This practice, simple but profoundly transformative, is a path to wholeness, connection and service to the greater good.

Chapter 16
Activation of the Light Body

The light body is an advanced energetic structure that connects the human being with higher dimensions of consciousness. It represents a vibrational vehicle that transcends the limits of the physical body and linear time, allowing the practitioner to access expanded states of healing, transformation, and spiritual connection. In the Arcturian holistic healing system, working with the light body not only raises the vibration of the practitioner but also opens doors to deep levels of self-knowledge and energetic service.

The Arcturians teach that the light body is present in all beings, although it is not always activated or fully functioning. Its activation requires a conscious alignment with high frequencies, as well as physical, mental, and spiritual preparation. Once activated, the light body becomes a channel to receive, integrate, and emit higher energies, facilitating deep healing and a direct connection with the Arcturian dimensions.

The first step in working with the light body is energetic preparation. This includes practices such as cleaning the auric field, harmonizing the chakras, and grounding. These techniques ensure that the energy system is in balance and ready to receive the frequencies needed to activate the light body.

One of the most common techniques for accessing the light body is visualization. During meditation, the practitioner can imagine a three-dimensional geometric structure, such as a Merkaba, rotating around them. This pattern, composed of two intertwined tetrahedrons rotating in opposite directions, represents the union of the physical and spiritual body. As the practitioner visualizes this form, they can imagine energy flowing through it, activating every cell and every part of their energy field.

Conscious breathing is also a powerful tool in this process. By inhaling deeply, the practitioner can visualize golden or silver light entering their body, filling every corner of their being. When exhaling, they can imagine this light expanding outward, forming a vibrant sphere that represents their light body. This breathing cycle not only activates the light body but also strengthens its connection to the higher dimensions.

Sound is another key technique for working with the light body. Specific tones, such as chanting "OM" or frequencies generated by crystal bowls, resonate directly with the vibrational structure of the light body, facilitating its activation and stabilization. During a session, the practitioner can use these sounds while visualizing the light body, allowing the vibrations to penetrate deeply into their system.

Working with Arcturian sacred symbols is also fundamental to accessing the light body. These symbols act as vibrational keys that unlock and activate different aspects of the energy body. For example, the Flower of Life symbol can be visualized rotating around the practitioner's body, harmonizing and strengthening their energy structure while connecting with higher frequencies.

Conscious physical movement, such as yoga or specific exercises designed to activate the energy body, also plays an important role. Gentle movements, combined with breathing and visualization, help to unblock stagnant areas and integrate the energies needed to activate the light body. The Arcturians recommend movements that mimic natural patterns, such as spirals or spins, to synchronize the physical body with the energy flow.

Once activated, the light body becomes a tool for exploring higher dimensions and working with more advanced energies. During meditation, the practitioner can use their light body to travel to high vibrational spaces, where they can receive guidance, healing, or information about their spiritual path. This process does not imply a disconnection from the physical body, but rather an expansion of consciousness that transcends the limits of time and space.

Access to the light body also allows the practitioner to channel higher energies more efficiently. In healing sessions, the light body acts as a conduit for Arcturian frequencies, amplifying their impact and allowing a deeper connection with the recipient. This approach not only strengthens the practitioner's energy field but also raises the vibration of the environment and those who interact with it.

As the practitioner works with their light body, it is important to integrate the experiences and balance the energies. The Arcturians teach that after each practice, the practitioner should take time to reconnect with the Earth, using grounding techniques such as walking barefoot or meditating on the root chakra. This ensures that the higher frequencies integrate harmoniously into the energy system, preventing imbalances or overloads.

Working with the light body not only transforms the practitioner but also has an impact on the collective energy field. By activating and strengthening this vibrational structure, the practitioner radiates higher frequencies that benefit their surroundings and contribute to planetary balance. This act of energetic service is a tangible expression of universal interconnection, reminding the practitioner of their role in collective evolution.

The Arcturians remind us that access to the light body is a gradual and continuous process. It is not about achieving an ideal state, but rather about exploring and deepening the connection with this vibrational structure with each practice. Through constancy and conscious intention, the practitioner not only transforms their energetic experience but also becomes a clear and powerful channel for higher energies.

The light body is a reminder of our multidimensional nature and our potential to transcend the limits of the physical. By working with it, the practitioner not only accesses higher states of consciousness but also contributes to the creation of a more harmonious and vibrant world, in tune with the higher frequencies of the universe.

Reconnection with the essence is a return to the deepest core of being, a process of remembering who we truly are, beyond the layers of accumulated experiences, beliefs, and emotions. In the Arcturian holistic healing system, this practice represents a return to the true nature of the practitioner: a vibrational and multidimensional being, connected to universal frequencies and unconditional love.

The Arcturians teach that the essence of each individual is a divine spark, a pure extension of universal energy. However, the dynamics of everyday life, dense emotions, and mental patterns can obscure this connection, creating a sense of separation and disconnection. Reconnection with the essence not only restores this connection but also allows the practitioner to access their inner power and unlimited capacity to heal and manifest.

The first step in this process is conscious self-observation. The practitioner must dedicate time to explore their thoughts, emotions, and beliefs without judgment, simply recognizing them as part of their human experience. This practice creates an inner space of acceptance that allows for the release of superficial layers and a closer approach to the core of one's being.

A powerful tool for reconnecting with the essence is meditation. During this practice, the practitioner can visualize a bright light in the center of their chest, representing their divine spark. As they focus on this light, they can imagine it slowly expanding, filling their entire body and energy field. This symbolic act not only reinforces the connection with the essence but also cleanses and revitalizes the energy system.

Conscious breathing is another essential technique. When inhaling, the practitioner can visualize bringing pure energy and high vibrations into their body. When exhaling, they can imagine releasing any energy or thought that separates them from their essence. This constant flow of conscious breathing acts as a vibrational bridge between the practitioner and their inner core.

The use of Arcturian frequencies is key in reconnecting with the essence. During a healing session or meditation, the practitioner can invoke these higher energies, visualizing them flowing into their body like a ray of golden or blue light. These frequencies work directly on the energy field, clearing blockages and restoring the connection with the divine essence.

Sacred symbols can also be used to deepen this practice. The Arcturians teach that certain geometric patterns, such as the Flower of Life or Metatron's Cube, resonate with the vibration of essence. By visualizing or drawing these symbols, the practitioner activates these frequencies in their energy system, reinforcing the connection with their inner core.

Nature is an invaluable ally in the reconnection process. Spending time outdoors, especially in quiet and natural environments, helps the practitioner clear their mind and tune into the universal flow. Walking barefoot on the earth, observing the sky, or simply sitting by a tree can be simple but profoundly transformative acts that facilitate reconnection with essence.

Working with the heart is central to this practice. The Arcturians teach that the heart is the portal to essence, the place where the purest vibrations of love and compassion are found. The practitioner can focus on their heart chakra, visualizing a warm light emanating from this center and connecting them with their essence. Repeating affirmations such as "I am connected to my divine essence" or "I live from my truth" can amplify this connection.

Introspective writing is another valuable tool for exploring and reconnecting with essence. By writing about questions such as "What am I really?" or "What connects me to my true nature?", the practitioner opens a space to reflect and receive intuitive impressions. This practice not only helps to release superficial layers but also offers clarity on the path to essence.

Reconnection with essence is not just an internal process, but also a life practice. The Arcturians remind us that every choice, thought, and action can align with our deepest truth. By living from essence, the practitioner experiences greater clarity, purpose, and fluidity in all areas of their life.

The impact of this reconnection transcends the individual. When the practitioner lives from their essence, they radiate a high energy that influences their surroundings and those around them. This vibration not only inspires others to reconnect with their own essence but also contributes to the balance and evolution of the collective energy field.

As the practitioner deepens this practice, they may experience a complete transformation in their perception of themselves and the universe. Separation gives way to unity, fear dissolves into love, and doubt is replaced by an unshakeable trust in their divine nature.

Reconnection with essence is a reminder that, at the core of our existence, we are beings of light and love, connected with universal frequencies. By returning to this truth, the practitioner not only finds peace and fulfillment but also discovers their unlimited capacity to heal, transform, and manifest a world in harmony with their divine essence.

Chapter 17
Reprogramming and Interdimensional Healing

Energy reprogramming is a profound and transformative practice within the Arcturian holistic healing system, designed to identify and transmute dysfunctional energy patterns that may have taken root in the energy system. These patterns, which often originate in limiting beliefs, past traumas, or external influences, not only affect emotional and mental well-being but also interfere with the natural flow of higher energies.

The Arcturians teach that energy reprogramming does not imply a rejection of these patterns, but an understanding of their origin and purpose, followed by a conscious process of release and transformation. Through this practice, the practitioner not only eliminates blockages but also creates a space for the integration of higher frequencies and more harmonious vibrations.

The first step in energy reprogramming is the conscious identification of the patterns that need to be transformed. This requires sincere and non-judgmental self-observation, in which the practitioner reflects on areas of their life where they feel resistance, stagnation, or repetition of negative experiences. Questions such as "What beliefs are limiting me?" or "What patterns do I keep repeating in my relationships or decisions?" can be helpful to begin this process.

A powerful tool for this phase is introspective writing. By taking the time to write about recurring thoughts, difficult emotions, or challenging experiences, the practitioner can begin to identify the underlying patterns that are affecting their energy system. This practice not only offers clarity but also acts as a first step in releasing these energies.

Once a pattern is identified, the next step is to connect with Arcturian frequencies to facilitate its transformation. During a meditation, the practitioner can visualize a ray of golden light descending towards their energy system, illuminating and enveloping the identified pattern. This light not only dissolves the dense energies associated with the pattern but also introduces new frequencies that support a higher and more harmonious state.

The use of affirmations is another central technique in energy reprogramming. Affirmations are conscious statements that act as vibrational seeds, replacing limiting patterns with more expansive beliefs. For example, if the practitioner has identified a pattern of insecurity, they can repeat affirmations such as "I trust my ability to navigate life with confidence" or "I am aligned with my inner power." Repeating these affirmations regularly, especially during meditations or before sleep, amplifies their impact.

Guided visualization is a powerful tool for reprogramming the energy system. The practitioner can imagine that the identified pattern is represented as a specific shape or color in their body or energy field. Then, they can visualize this pattern gradually dissolving, transforming into light or a higher frequency. This process not only releases blocked energy but also establishes a new vibrational flow in the system.

Sound is another effective vibrational technique for energy reprogramming. Chanting mantras, specific tones, or using instruments such as Tibetan bowls or bells generates frequencies that resonate deeply within the energy system, helping to release and reconfigure limiting patterns. For example, the sound "OM" is ideal for balancing and harmonizing the system, preparing the energy field to integrate new vibrations.

Working with crystals can complement these techniques. Stones such as amethyst, rose quartz, or obsidian have specific properties that help release dense patterns and anchor new frequencies. Placing a crystal on the area of the body where the pattern is perceived, or holding it while repeating affirmations, amplifies the reprogramming process.

The physical body also plays an important role in energy reprogramming. The Arcturians teach that many energy patterns manifest as physical tension or blockages. Practices such as yoga, tai chi, or intuitive movement help release these tensions and restore the natural flow of energy in the body. Conscious movements, combined with deep breathing and visualization, enhance this effect.

Once the pattern has been released, it is crucial to establish a clear intention for the new energy flow. This can be achieved by visualizing an ideal state of balance and well-being, or imagining how the practitioner interacts with the world from a place of empowerment and clarity. This act of conscious creation ensures that the energy system reconfigures itself in a way that is aligned with the practitioner's highest intentions.

Integration is an essential part of energy reprogramming. After working with a pattern, the practitioner should take time to rest, reflect, and allow the new frequencies to settle into their system. The Arcturians emphasize the importance of connecting with the earth during this stage, using practices such as walking barefoot on the ground or meditating with the root chakra to stabilize the energies.

The impact of energy reprogramming is not limited to the practitioner. As they release limiting patterns and raise their vibration, they also radiate these frequencies to their surroundings, contributing to the collective balance. This process is an act of healing not only personal, but also universal, reminding the practitioner of their interconnectedness with the whole.

The Arcturians teach us that energy reprogramming is a continuous journey, an opportunity to explore, release, and transform the energies that have shaped us. Through this practice, the practitioner not only discovers their power to change their reality, but also aligns with their deepest truth, creating a path to wholeness and spiritual expansion.

Interdimensional healing is an advanced practice within the Arcturian holistic healing system that transcends the limitations of the physical plane to address energy imbalances in higher dimensions. The Arcturians teach that blockages and dysfunctional patterns often have roots that go beyond the present experience, originating in other dimensions, past lives, or parallel timelines. This approach allows the practitioner to work with these energies at a deeper level, promoting complete and lasting healing.

The fundamental principle of interdimensional healing is the understanding that all dimensions are interconnected through a universal energy field. By consciously accessing this field, the practitioner can identify and transform energies that affect the present system, restoring balance at all levels of being. This process not only raises the recipient's vibration but also facilitates their alignment with their highest purpose.

To initiate an interdimensional healing practice, it is crucial to prepare the practitioner's energy space. This includes grounding techniques, clearing the auric field, and aligning with higher frequencies. The Arcturians emphasize the importance of creating a sacred space, both physical and energetic, that provides protection and focus during the session.

Meditation is an essential tool for accessing higher dimensions. The practitioner can visualize a portal of bright light in front of them, representing the entrance to interdimensional levels. Upon crossing this portal, they can feel their energy field expand, connecting with a network of higher vibrations. During this process, it is essential to establish a clear intention, such as "I access the higher dimensions to facilitate healing in alignment with the highest good."

Intuition plays a crucial role in interdimensional healing. As the practitioner explores these dimensions, they may receive impressions in the form of images, sounds, sensations, or simply intuitive knowledge. These perceptions offer clues about the imbalances present and the energies that need attention. For example, the practitioner may perceive an energy blockage as a shadow, a knot, or a repetitive pattern, indicating an area that requires healing.

Working with Arcturian frequencies is central to this practice. During the session, the practitioner can visualize rays of golden, blue, or violet light flowing to the identified area, dissolving blockages and restoring energy flow. These frequencies act as catalysts that not only cleanse but also reconfigure the recipient's vibration in alignment with their higher essence.

Sacred geometry is another powerful tool in interdimensional healing. The Arcturians teach that certain geometric patterns, such as the Merkabah or the Star Tetrahedron, resonate with the higher dimensions and facilitate access to them. During a session, the practitioner can visualize these patterns rotating and expanding around the recipient, balancing their energy system and connecting them with their multidimensional being.

Time and space are flexible concepts in interdimensional work. Energy blockages can originate in past lives, potential futures, or parallel timelines. By accessing these levels, the practitioner can identify events or experiences that have left an energetic mark and work to release them. This process does not alter the events themselves, but transforms how their energies affect the recipient in the present.

Sound is an effective vibrational tool in this practice. Chanting specific mantras, such as "OM" or channeled Arcturian tones, helps synchronize the practitioner with higher frequencies. Instruments such as crystal bowls or tuning forks can also be used to generate vibrations that resonate with interdimensional dimensions, amplifying healing.

Energy protection is crucial during interdimensional healing. Before beginning, the practitioner can visualize a sphere of white or golden light around them, acting as a shield that allows only the highest and purest energies. In addition, invoking Arcturian guides or spiritual masters ensures that the session is conducted in a space of safety and clarity.

Upon concluding the session, it is important to consciously close the interdimensional work. The practitioner can visualize the portal of light gently closing, sealing the energies worked with and ensuring that the recipient remains balanced and protected. It is also recommended to perform a grounding to integrate the transformed energies into the physical plane.

The effects of interdimensional healing are profound and multifaceted. The recipient not only experiences relief from blockages or imbalances but may also feel greater clarity, peace, and connection to their higher purpose. This work also positively impacts the collective energy field, contributing to planetary and universal balance.

The Arcturians teach that interdimensional healing is a reminder of our multidimensional nature and our ability to transform the energies that affect our present experience. As the practitioner deepens this practice, they not only expand their understanding of the energetic universe but also become a more powerful channel for higher frequencies, bringing light and harmony to all levels of existence.

This work is both an art and a spiritual science, an invitation to explore the infinite possibilities of healing and transformation from the highest dimensions to the physical plane. Interdimensional healing not only connects the practitioner with the universe, but also reminds them that they are an integral and active part of its energetic fabric.

Chapter 18
Arcturian Masters and Symbols

In the Arcturian holistic healing system, working with masters is a profoundly transformative practice that connects the practitioner with spiritual guides and high-vibrational beings. Arcturian masters, like other multidimensional guides, act as allies in the healing process, providing guidance, energy, and support at the highest levels of consciousness. This work strengthens the practitioner's spiritual connection, raises their vibration, and expands their ability to channel and direct higher energies.

The Arcturians teach that the masters are always available to offer their assistance, but conscious connection requires intention and openness on the part of the practitioner. Working with these guides is not based on a passive act of receiving, but on an active and respectful collaboration that recognizes the autonomy and inner power of the practitioner.

The first step in working with masters is to establish a clear intention. The practitioner can formulate a specific request, such as "I seek the guidance of the Arcturian masters to heal this blockage" or "I invoke the presence of my guides to receive guidance in this challenge." This intention not only acts as a vibrational bridge, but also ensures that the connection takes place in alignment with the practitioner's highest good.

Energetic preparation is essential before starting a practice with masters. This includes cleansing the auric field, balancing the chakras, and grounding. Creating a sacred space, both physical and energetic, is also important. This can be done by lighting candles, using crystals, placing sacred symbols, or playing high-frequency music to raise the vibration of the environment.

Meditation is one of the most effective tools for establishing contact with masters. During this practice, the practitioner can visualize a bright light descending from the higher dimensions towards their crown, filling them with a sense of peace and clarity. While immersed in this state, they can imagine the presence of the Arcturian masters or other guides, feeling their energy and opening themselves to their communication.

Communication with masters can manifest in different ways, depending on the sensitivity and intuitive channel of the practitioner. Some people may receive messages in the form of words or phrases, while others experience images, physical sensations, or simply intuitive knowing. It is important to trust these perceptions, even if they seem subtle or vague at first, as with practice they become clearer and more consistent.

Arcturian sacred symbols are powerful tools for working with masters. Each symbol contains a specific frequency that facilitates connection with these beings of light. During a session, the practitioner can visualize a symbol floating in front of them or trace it with their hands in the energy space. This act not only establishes a vibrational bridge, but also amplifies the reception of energy and guidance from the masters.

The use of sound is another effective technique for strengthening the connection with the masters. Chanting mantras, such as "OM" or channeled Arcturian tones, generates a vibration that resonates with the higher dimensions. Instruments such as crystal bowls or bells can also be used to raise the frequency of the practitioner and the space, facilitating communication with the guides.

Channeled writing is an advanced practice that allows you to receive direct messages from the masters. During a meditation, the practitioner can have paper and pen at hand, allowing the words to flow without filtering or analyzing. This process not only provides clear guidance, but also acts as a tangible record of interaction with the masters.

Working with masters is not limited to receiving messages, but also includes collaboration in healing practices. During a session, the practitioner can invoke the masters to channel energy to the recipient or guide the direction of the session. This collaboration not only enhances healing, but also raises the vibration of the practitioner and strengthens their confidence in their abilities.

It is important that the practitioner develops discernment in working with masters. Although these guides operate from high frequencies, the practitioner must trust their intuition to ensure that the connection is made with beings aligned with love and light. The Arcturians teach that any message or energy that generates fear, confusion, or doubt does not come from a true master, and should be released with gratitude and firmness.

When finishing a practice, it is essential to express gratitude to the masters for their guidance and support. This act not only reinforces the vibrational connection, but also maintains a balanced flow of energy between the practitioner and the guides. Furthermore, consciously closing the session ensures that the practitioner returns to their physical state fully present and grounded.

The benefits of working with masters are profound and multifaceted. In addition to receiving guidance and healing, the practitioner develops a deeper connection with their own higher self and with the higher dimensions. This work also strengthens the practitioner's confidence, clarity, and ability to act as a conscious channel of light and love.

The Arcturians remind us that working with masters is an expression of universal interconnectedness. By collaborating with these guides, the practitioner not only raises their own vibration, but also contributes to the balance and evolution of the collective energy field. This process is a reminder that we are never alone on our path, but that we are always surrounded by beings who wish to support and guide us towards our highest expression.

Working with masters is an invitation to explore the depth of our spiritual connection and to remember our ability to interact with the universe from a place of love, trust, and clarity. Through this practice, the practitioner not only transforms their own experience, but also becomes a beacon of light for those around them, radiating the highest frequencies of harmony and healing.

Arcturian symbols are vibrational portals that connect the practitioner with higher energies, facilitating healing, harmonization, and spiritual expansion. These sacred patterns, transmitted from higher dimensions, not only contain specific frequencies, but also act as energy maps that guide the flow of energy in the recipient's system. In the Arcturian holistic healing system, the conscious use of these symbols allows unlocking latent potentials, transmuting densities, and strengthening the connection with the higher dimensions.

The Arcturians teach that each symbol has a unique energetic signature, designed to interact with specific aspects of the human energy field. Some symbols promote cleansing and protection, while others activate the light body, balance the chakras, or strengthen the connection to the higher self. By working with these symbols, the practitioner not only channels the associated energies, but also raises their own vibration by aligning with the higher frequencies they represent.

The first step in working with Arcturian symbols is to become familiar with their energy and meaning. Although some symbols may be transmitted through specific teachings, many practitioners discover new patterns intuitively during meditations or channeling. It is essential to approach this process with openness and respect, recognizing that each symbol is a sacred tool that should be used with clear intention and aligned with the highest good.

Activating a symbol is essential to unlock its vibrational potential. This can be done by visualizing the symbol floating in front of the practitioner or tracing it with their hands in the air. While activating it, the practitioner sets a clear intention that guides the purpose of the symbol, such as "This symbol activates the harmonization of my energy field" or "This pattern strengthens my connection to the higher dimensions."

During a healing session, symbols can be applied directly to the recipient's energy field. For example, a cleansing symbol can be visualized over the root chakra to release blockages, while an activation pattern can be placed on the third eye to stimulate intuition. The Arcturians teach that the practitioner's intention, combined with the energy of the symbol, is what creates the vibrational impact on the recipient.

The use of symbols in combination with other tools, such as crystals or sound, enhances their effectiveness. For example, a protection symbol can be traced while using a clear quartz to seal the recipient's energy field, or an activation pattern can be combined with the sound of a Tibetan bowl to enhance its resonance. These combinations not only intensify the flow of energy, but also create a more complete and harmonious healing experience.

Symbols can also be integrated into meditations and visualizations. During a meditative practice, the practitioner can imagine themselves surrounded by a specific geometric pattern, allowing its energy to permeate their entire energy field. This visualization not only strengthens the connection with the higher frequencies, but also acts as a deep cleansing and harmonization of the system.

In space healing, Arcturian symbols are valuable tools for raising the vibration of an environment. A practitioner can trace a cleansing symbol in the corners of a room, or place physical representations of the patterns at strategic points to maintain energy balance. This practice is especially useful in places where dense energies or frequent imbalances are perceived.

The use of symbols is not limited to direct energy work. They can also be incorporated into art, writing, or as part of altars and sacred spaces. For example, a practitioner may draw a symbol in a journal as part of a specific intention, or use it as a talisman to carry with them throughout the day. These simple acts keep the practitioner connected to the frequencies of the symbol and reinforce its impact on daily life.

The intuitive creation of new symbols is an advanced practice in the Arcturian system. Practitioners who have developed a deep connection with the higher dimensions may receive unique patterns during meditations or channeling. These symbols, although personal in origin, contain universal frequencies that can be shared and applied in healing or spiritual development contexts.

It is important to remember that working with Arcturian symbols requires respect and responsibility. The Arcturians teach that these patterns are not tools to manipulate or impose energies, but means to collaborate with higher frequencies for the benefit of the practitioner and the collective. Using them with a pure and ethical intention ensures that their impact is positive and transformative.

The impact of Arcturian symbols is profound and multifaceted. By working with them, the practitioner not only accesses high levels of healing and spiritual connection, but also contributes to the energy balance of the environment and to collective well-being. These patterns act as tangible reminders of universal interconnectedness and the vibrational potential that resides in each being.

The Arcturians remind us that symbols are not just external tools, but also representations of energies that already exist within us. By working with these patterns, the practitioner not only channels higher frequencies, but also activates latent aspects of their own energy, remembering their innate ability to heal, transform, and manifest harmony.

Working with Arcturian symbols is an invitation to explore the depths of the vibrational universe and discover new ways to collaborate with higher energies. Through this practice, the practitioner not only raises their own vibration, but also becomes a bridge between dimensions, radiating light and balance to the world around them.

Chapter 19
Reconstruction of Energetic DNA and Ancestral Healing

The reconstruction of energetic DNA is an advanced practice in the Arcturian holistic healing system that seeks to restore and activate the highest frequencies encoded in the subtle DNA. This DNA does not refer solely to the physical structure we know, but to an energetic pattern that contains the memory and vibrational potential of our multidimensional essence. The Arcturians teach that by working with energetic DNA, it is possible to release deep blockages, activate latent capacities, and align the practitioner with their higher purpose.

Energetic DNA is a bridge between the physical body and the higher dimensions, a matrix that holds information not only from this life, but from past lives, parallel timelines, and the future potential of the being. However, factors such as traumas, limiting beliefs, and dense energies can distort this pattern, preventing it from manifesting in its fullness. The reconstruction of energetic DNA allows for the elimination of these distortions, restoring its original vibration and unlocking higher levels of consciousness and healing.

The first step in this practice is to consciously connect with the energetic DNA. This begins with a guided meditation in which the practitioner visualizes a golden helix of light that represents their energetic DNA. As they focus on this image, they can imagine that the light begins to expand, enveloping their entire energy field and awakening latent frequencies.

Conscious breathing is a fundamental tool for working with energetic DNA. During practice, the practitioner can inhale deeply, imagining that the golden light flows into their system, cleansing and revitalizing each fiber of their energetic DNA. Upon exhaling, they can visualize releasing any energy or pattern that distorts this vibrational flow. This breathing cycle not only strengthens the connection but also activates the reconstruction process.

The use of Arcturian frequencies is essential in this practice. The Arcturians teach that certain vibrations, such as violet and golden light, resonate directly with energetic DNA, facilitating its repair and activation. During a session, the practitioner can visualize a beam of Arcturian light flowing into their DNA, repairing any interruption in their energy pattern and activating their highest potential.

Sacred geometry also plays a fundamental role in the reconstruction of energetic DNA. Patterns such as the Flower of Life or Metatron's Cube can be visualized rotating around the energy helix, stabilizing its structure and aligning it with higher frequencies. These patterns act as matrices of perfection that guide the energy flow to an ideal state.

Specific sounds and mantras are vibrational tools that amplify the impact of this practice. Chanting sacred tones, such as "RA" or "OM", or the use of crystal bowls at high frequencies, generates a resonance that penetrates deeply into the energetic DNA system. These sounds not only clear distortions but also awaken dormant codes that contain ancestral wisdom and spiritual capacities.

Working with crystals is another important component. Crystals such as selenite, clear quartz, and labradorite resonate directly with the frequencies of energetic DNA. During a session, the practitioner can place these crystals at strategic points on the body, such as the crown chakra or solar plexus, to amplify energy flow and stabilize the reconstruction process.

Channeled writing can also be helpful for working with energetic DNA. During a meditation, the practitioner can allow words or symbols to flow that represent the vibrational patterns of their DNA. Writing these messages not only helps to integrate the process, but also acts as a tangible reminder of the activated energies.

The reconstruction of energetic DNA is not an immediate process, but a gradual path that requires patience and dedication. The Arcturians emphasize that each practice deepens the connection with the energy pattern, releasing layers of density and activating new frequencies. This work can bring about significant changes in the practitioner's perception, intuition, and overall well-being.

Furthermore, this process has an impact that goes beyond the individual. As the practitioner reconstructs and activates their energetic DNA, they radiate higher frequencies to their surroundings, contributing to collective balance and planetary well-being. This work is a reminder that personal transformation and collective evolution are intrinsically connected.

Integration is a crucial part of this practice. After working with energetic DNA, the practitioner should take time to rest, hydrate, and connect with the Earth. This ensures that the new frequencies settle harmoniously in their system and that the activation process continues even after the session.

The reconstruction of energetic DNA is an invitation to remember our true nature as multidimensional beings and access our unlimited potential. Through this practice, the practitioner not only transforms their own experience but also contributes to the creation of a more harmonious and vibrant world, in alignment with the higher frequencies of the universe.

The Arcturians remind us that working with energetic DNA is an act of love and self-discovery. Each activated energy fiber is a step towards a greater connection with the higher self and with the universal flow. This deeply transformative practice is a path to wholeness, healing, and spiritual expansion.

Ancestral healing is a powerful practice in the Arcturian holistic healing system that addresses the energetic and emotional patterns inherited through generations. The Arcturians teach that the experiences, beliefs, and traumas of our ancestors remain not only in genetic memory, but also in the energy fields of their descendants, influencing their physical, emotional, and spiritual well-being. Healing these inherited energies not only frees the individual but also transforms the entire lineage and contributes to collective balance.

The foundation of ancestral healing lies in the interconnection of souls within a lineage. Each member of a lineage shares a common energy field that contains both wisdom and gifts as well as wounds and blockages. These energies can manifest as repetitive patterns in relationships, health, or life circumstances, signaling the need to heal and release.

The first step in this practice is to acknowledge and honor the connection with ancestors. Before beginning any energy work, the practitioner can take a moment to express gratitude to their ancestors, recognizing their sacrifices, their achievements, and their influence on their own existence. This act of respect creates a sacred space for healing and reinforces the intention to work in alignment with the highest good of the entire lineage.

Meditation is a key tool for connecting with ancestral energies. During a meditative practice, the practitioner can visualize a chain of light extending back in time, representing each of their ancestors. As they focus on this chain, they can invoke the Arcturian guides to accompany them in the process, providing clarity, protection, and energetic support.

The use of specific Arcturian symbols amplifies ancestral healing. For example, a release symbol can be visualized floating above the ancestral chain, dissolving dense patterns and allowing the flow of energy to return to its natural state. These symbols not only clear inherited energies but also activate frequencies that strengthen the positive aspects of the lineage.

Working with vibrational frequency is another fundamental technique. During a session, the practitioner can imagine that a beam of golden light flows from the higher dimensions to the ancestral chain, clearing blockages and restoring balance. This light acts as a catalyst, transmuting dense energies into high and harmonious vibrations.

Introspective writing can also be a useful tool for exploring ancestral patterns. By reflecting on questions such as "What patterns do I observe in my family that I wish to transform?" or "What emotional legacy do I feel I carry?", the practitioner can identify specific areas that need attention. This practice not only provides clarity but also opens a channel of communication with ancestral energies.

Crystals are powerful allies in ancestral healing. Stones such as amethyst, obsidian, and labradorite resonate with frequencies that help release inherited patterns and protect the practitioner's energy field. During a session, these crystals can be placed on the root chakra or on an altar dedicated to ancestors, amplifying the impact of the practice.

Sound is another vibrational tool that facilitates ancestral healing. Chanting mantras, using drums, or playing Tibetan bowls generates frequencies that resonate deeply with inherited energies, helping to release blockages and restore balance. For example, the drum, with its constant rhythm, can act as a vibrational bridge that connects the practitioner to the roots of their lineage.

Forgiveness is an essential component of ancestral healing. Many of the inherited patterns are linked to emotional wounds that need to be released. During a session, the practitioner can visualize sending light and compassion to the ancestors associated with these wounds, expressing intentions of forgiveness and release. This act not only relieves the burden of the lineage but also frees the practitioner from the associated energetic burdens.

Integrating ancestral gifts is as important as releasing dense patterns. The Arcturians teach that each lineage has unique wisdom, strengths, and qualities that can be activated and honored. During a meditation, the practitioner can visualize receiving these positive energies, integrating them into their energy field as a resource for their daily life.

Ancestral healing not only benefits the practitioner but also radiates to future generations. By releasing inherited patterns, the practitioner interrupts dysfunctional energy cycles, creating a space for their descendants to live in greater balance and harmony. This work is a gift to the entire lineage, an act of service that transcends time and space.

The Arcturians remind us that ancestral healing is an ongoing process, a path of release and connection that requires patience and compassion. Each practice deepens the practitioner's relationship with their lineage and strengthens their connection with universal energies.

Ultimately, ancestral healing is an act of love and reconciliation, an opportunity to transform inherited energies into a source of strength and wisdom. Through this practice, the practitioner not only honors their ancestors, but also becomes a bridge between the past and the future, radiating light and balance to all generations of their lineage.

Chapter 20
Sound and Heart Healing

Sound is one of the most powerful tools in the Arcturian holistic healing system, a vibrational vehicle capable of penetrating deeply into the energy field and reconfiguring it at the cellular and multidimensional levels. Integrating sound into healing practices allows for the unblocking of stagnant energy, restoring vibrational balance, and facilitating connections with higher frequencies. The Arcturians teach that sound, when used with conscious intention, is a direct bridge to healing and transformation.

Each sound generates a vibration that interacts with the physical, emotional, and energetic body. Harmonic frequencies have the power to dissolve blockages, activate energy centers, and align the practitioner with their higher self. This unique ability makes sound a versatile and effective tool at any stage of the healing process.

The first step in working with sound is to understand its impact on the energy system. Low, deep tones, such as those generated by drums or large Tibetan bowls, resonate with the lower chakras, promoting grounding and stability. On the other hand, higher tones, such as those produced by crystal bowls or bells, stimulate the upper chakras, facilitating mental clarity and spiritual expansion.

Breathing is a key component in sound integration. Before using any vibrational tool, the practitioner can take deep breaths to tune into their own energy flow. While inhaling, they can imagine the sound beginning to resonate in their field, preparing their system to receive the frequencies. When exhaling, they can visualize releasing blockages or tensions, allowing the sound to work more effectively.

One of the most common tools in sound healing is the use of Tibetan and crystal bowls. These instruments generate pure tones that penetrate deep into the body and energy field, promoting a state of relaxation and balance. During a session, the practitioner can play a bowl near the recipient, allowing the sound waves to interact directly with their energy system.

Chanting mantras is another powerful technique for integrating sound into healing. Mantras are vibrational formulas that contain specific frequencies designed to harmonize the energy system. For example, the mantra "OM" resonates with the universal frequency, creating a sense of unity and connection. By repeating a mantra, the practitioner not only works with the external sound but also with the internal vibration of their own voice, amplifying its impact.

The shamanic drum is an ancestral tool that is also used in Arcturian practices. Its constant and deep rhythm resonates with the heartbeat, creating a stabilizing effect on the energy field. During a session, the drum can be played near specific areas of the body or in a rhythmic pattern that invites energy to move and flow.

The use of tuning forks is a more precise technique within sound healing. These instruments generate specific frequencies that can be applied directly to energy points or chakras. For example, a tuning fork tuned to a frequency related to the heart chakra can be placed over this center, allowing the vibration to penetrate deeply and promote its balance.

High-frequency music is another useful tool for integrating sound into healing practices. Pieces designed with frequencies like 432 Hz or 528 Hz have specific properties that facilitate relaxation, harmonization, and healing. These frequencies can be played in the background during a session or listened to in personal meditations to strengthen the connection with higher energies.

Sound acts not only on the recipient but also on the space where the practice is performed. The Arcturians teach that sound cleanses and raises the vibration of the environment, creating a sacred space where energies can flow freely. Playing instruments such as bells or chimes in the corners of a room is an effective way to prepare the space before a healing session.

Integrating sound into visualizations amplifies its vibrational impact. During a meditation, the practitioner can imagine a sacred geometric pattern, such as the Flower of Life, vibrating to the rhythm of a specific sound. This combination not only intensifies the experience but also enhances the harmonization and activation of the energy field.

The use of sound in healing is not limited to external instruments or techniques. The practitioner's voice is a powerful tool in itself, capable of channeling high frequencies to the recipient. The Arcturians teach that singing, humming, or even emitting intuitive sounds during a session acts as a direct channel of higher energies, adapting to the specific needs of the recipient.

Integrating sound into healing practices also requires conscious closure. After working with intense frequencies, the practitioner can play a soft instrument or sing a calming mantra to stabilize the recipient's energy field. This act not only ensures a harmonious transition but also seals the energies worked with, allowing the effects of healing to integrate in a deep and lasting way.

Sound is a vibrational expression of the universe, a reminder of our connection to all that exists. By integrating it into healing practices, the practitioner not only transforms their own energy field but also contributes to the balance and harmony of the collective. This vibrational tool, used with intention and awareness, is a path to healing and ascension.

The heart is the energy center where the physical, emotional, mental, and spiritual dimensions converge. It is the place where the capacity to experience unconditional love, compassion, and connection with all that exists resides. In the Arcturian holistic healing system, heart healing is a central practice that allows for the release of emotional blockages, the restoration of inner harmony, and the unlocking of the natural flow of energy in the vibrational field.

The Arcturians teach that the heart chakra, or Anahata, acts as a bridge between the lower chakras, which focus on connection to the Earth and physical needs, and the higher chakras, which promote spiritual expansion and connection to higher dimensions. For this reason, heart healing not only transforms emotional well-being but also strengthens balance and energetic alignment at all levels.

The first step in heart healing is to create a safe space for emotional exploration and release. This can be achieved through preparatory practices such as cleansing the energy field, using specific crystals, and creating a peaceful and harmonious environment. The Arcturians recommend elements such as rose quartz, warm light candles, and soft music to raise the vibration of the space.

Conscious self-observation is a key tool for identifying emotional blockages associated with the heart. The practitioner can reflect on recurring patterns of sadness, fear, or resentment that may be affecting their ability to give and receive love. These emotions, although often painful, are portals to transformation and release.

An essential technique for working with the heart is conscious breathing directed towards the center of the chest. During this practice, the practitioner can imagine that each inhalation brings green or pink light to the heart chakra, filling it with vibrant, healing energy. With each exhalation, they can visualize releasing any density or blockage, allowing the energy flow to be restored.

The use of Arcturian frequencies is fundamental in heart healing. During a meditation, the practitioner can visualize a ray of golden or emerald light descending from the higher dimensions to their heart chakra. This light works to dissolve emotional blockages, heal deep wounds, and activate the potential of unconditional love.

Sacred symbols are also powerful tools for heart healing. Patterns such as the Flower of Life or the Sacred Heart can be visualized gently rotating in the center of the chest, balancing and harmonizing energies. The Arcturians teach that these symbols act as vibrational portals, amplifying the impact of higher frequencies on the heart.

Sound is another vibrational tool that resonates deeply with the heart. Mantras, such as "YAM," associated with the heart chakra, or specific tones generated by Tibetan or crystal bowls, can be used during a healing session. These sounds not only unlock stagnant energies but also invite the vibration of love and compassion to flow freely.

Creative visualization is a transformative technique in this work. During a meditation, the practitioner can imagine an inner garden in their heart, full of light and vibrant colors. They can visualize this space flourishing with each breath, representing the expansion of love and inner healing. This process not only strengthens the connection with the heart but also provides a sense of peace and fulfillment.

Forgiveness is an essential component of heart healing. Many emotional wounds are linked to past events or difficult relationships. During a session, the practitioner can visualize sending light and compassion to these experiences, releasing them from their energy field. This act does not imply justifying past actions but releasing their emotional impact to restore inner balance.

Conscious physical contact can also support heart healing. Placing a hand over the center of the chest while repeating affirmations such as "I am open to unconditional love" or "My heart is in balance and harmony" amplifies the connection with this energy center. This simple gesture acts as a tangible reminder of the intention to heal and strengthen the heart.

Working with the heart not only benefits the practitioner but also radiates to their surroundings. The Arcturians teach that an open and balanced heart emits a high vibration that positively influences those around it, creating a collective healing effect. This impact is felt not only in personal relationships but also in the energetic balance of the collective.

Integration is a crucial step in heart healing. After working with this energy center, the practitioner should take time to reflect, rest, and allow the new energies to settle. Grounding practices, such as walking barefoot or meditating in contact with nature, help stabilize energy flow and integrate healing into daily life.

Heart healing is a continuous journey, an invitation to explore and embrace the essence of unconditional love that resides in each being. The

Arcturians remind us that this work not only transforms personal experience but also contributes to the balance and harmony of the world.

The heart, as a center of connection and compassion, is a reminder of our purest and most divine nature. By healing and activating this energy center, the practitioner not only releases their inner potential but also radiates light and love to everything around them, creating a profound and lasting impact on all levels of existence.

Chapter 21
Cosmic Alignment and Animal Healing

Planetary alignment is a fundamental concept within the Arcturian holistic healing system, which explores the relationship between planetary cycles and personal energetic well-being. The Arcturians teach that celestial bodies emit specific frequencies that influence not only the physical environment but also the vibrational field of human beings. By consciously working with these energies, the practitioner can attune themselves to universal rhythms, restore their inner balance, and enhance their connection to higher dimensions.

Planetary cycles are not just astronomical events; they represent energetic movements that affect collective and personal consciousness. For example, the Moon, with its cyclical influence, has a direct impact on emotions, while the transits of planets like Jupiter or Saturn can symbolize expansions or challenges in specific areas of life. Understanding these dynamics allows the practitioner to align their energy with these cosmic flows, harnessing their potential for healing and spiritual growth.

The first step in planetary alignment is the conscious observation of celestial cycles. This includes being aware of events such as full moons, eclipses, equinoxes, solstices, and major planetary transits. Each of these events has a unique energetic impact, which can be used to meditate, manifest intentions, or release emotional blockages.

The connection with the Moon is especially powerful in this practice. During the full moon, the practitioner can perform release rituals, letting go of dense energies or limiting patterns that no longer serve them. In contrast, the new moon is an ideal time to set intentions and sow new ideas. Visualizing the light of the Moon entering the practitioner's energy field can amplify these practices, harmonizing internal energies with lunar frequencies.

The Sun, as the main source of energy, also plays a crucial role in planetary alignment. During solstices and equinoxes, practitioners can work with the Sun's energy to balance their energy field. For example, at the summer solstice, one can channel solar frequencies to enhance vitality and growth, while at the winter solstice, introspection and energy restoration are the focus.

Conscious breathing and meditation are key tools for working with planetary energies. During a session, the practitioner can visualize a ray of light connecting their body with the corresponding planet or celestial cycle. For example, in a Venus transit, one can imagine a green or pink light, associated with love and connection, flowing into their heart chakra. This practice not only aligns the practitioner's energy with planetary frequencies but also activates the transformative potential of these influences.

The use of sacred geometry amplifies alignment with celestial cycles. During a practice, the practitioner can visualize geometric patterns such as the Flower of Life or the Merkaba rotating around their body, synchronizing with planetary energies. These patterns not only balance the energy field, but also create a vibrational bridge to universal rhythms.

Crystals are also valuable allies in planetary alignment. Stones such as labradorite, amethyst, and citrine resonate with specific celestial energies and can be used to amplify the connection to planetary cycles. Placing a crystal under the light of the full moon or near the practitioner during meditation enhances its vibration and facilitates attunement with cosmic energies.

Sound is another powerful tool for working with planetary alignment. Tibetan singing bowls, tuning forks, or even chanting specific mantras generate frequencies that resonate with celestial energies. For example, during an eclipse, playing a Tibetan singing bowl can help stabilize the energy field, allowing the practitioner to integrate the transformations associated with this event.

Intuitive writing and reflection are also useful practices during planetary cycles. By writing about the energies perceived during a celestial event or about the intentions one wishes to manifest, the practitioner anchors these energies in their conscious experience. This practice not only reinforces the connection with planetary rhythms but also provides clarity and purpose.

Planetary alignment has a profound impact on personal and collective well-being. By attuning to cosmic rhythms, the practitioner not only experiences greater inner harmony but also contributes to the energetic balance of their surroundings. This work is a reminder of the interconnection between human beings and the universe, an invitation to co-create with cosmic forces for well-being and spiritual expansion.

The Arcturians teach that planetary alignment is an act of balance and collaboration with the universe. By understanding and working with these energies, the practitioner not only strengthens their connection to the cosmos, but also accesses a vibrational flow that supports their personal and collective evolution.

This work not only transforms the practitioner, but also places them in sync with a greater purpose, reminding them that they are an integral part of a vast and dynamic universal fabric. Planetary alignment is a path to harmony, fulfillment, and spiritual expansion, a practice that connects the practitioner with the eternal rhythms of the cosmos.

Healing for animals is a practice deeply connected with Arcturian frequencies, designed to harmonize and restore the energetic balance of the beings that share the world with us. The Arcturians teach that animals are natural receivers and emitters of energy, and that their vibrational field is closely intertwined with that of humans and the Earth itself. Working with them from the perspective of healing not only benefits their well-being, but also strengthens the spiritual connection between species.

Animals, like humans, have energy fields that can become unbalanced due to external factors such as stress, the environment, or physical illness. However, their natural sensitivity to energies allows them to respond quickly to healing techniques, especially those that utilize high frequencies such as the Arcturian ones.

The first step in animal healing is preparing the energy space. Creating a calm, safe, and distraction-free environment is essential for the animal to feel comfortable and open to receiving energy. Using tools such as soft music, harmonizing crystals like rose quartz, or even natural scents like lavender can help raise the vibration of the environment.

Intuitive connection is essential in this practice. Before beginning, the practitioner should take a moment to tune in to the animal's energy, observing its body language, breathing, and behaviors. This act not only establishes a bond of trust, but also allows the practitioner to identify specific areas that need energetic attention.

The use of hands is a key technique in animal healing. The practitioner can place their hands a comfortable distance from the animal's body, allowing energy to flow naturally. During this process, one can visualize a ray of golden or green light emanating from the hands, enveloping the animal in a bubble of healing energy. It is important to observe the animal's responses, such as movements, relaxation, or changes in breathing, which indicate that it is absorbing the energy.

Arcturian frequencies are particularly effective in animal healing. During a session, the practitioner can invoke these higher energies, visualizing a flow of vibrant light connecting with the animal's energy field. This light not only works to release blockages or tensions, but also balances and strengthens their energy system.

Sound is another powerful tool in this practice. Gently playing a Tibetan singing bowl or chanting calming tones can generate vibrations that resonate with the animal's energy field, promoting relaxation and harmonization. For example, a cat may respond to a low tone with purring, while a dog may show signs of calmness and attention.

Crystals are also important allies in animal healing. Rose quartz, for example, resonates with energies of love and compassion, while amethyst promotes relaxation and peace. These crystals can be placed near the animal or held during a healing session to amplify the energy flow.

Conscious breathing is a technique that benefits both the practitioner and the animal. During a session, the practitioner can inhale deeply, imagining that they are absorbing healing energy from the higher dimensions. Upon exhaling, they can visualize this energy flowing to the animal, enveloping it in a mantle of vibrant light. This rhythmic flow of breath reinforces the energetic connection and amplifies the impact of healing.

Visualization is especially helpful when working with animals that are shy or uncomfortable with physical contact. In these cases, the practitioner can imagine the animal surrounded by a sphere of golden or green light, allowing energy to flow to it without the need for direct interaction. This approach is effective and respectful, especially for rescued animals or those with previous traumatic experiences.

Telepathic communication is an advanced skill in animal healing. As the practitioner develops their intuition, they may perceive impressions or messages from the animal, related to their needs or emotions. These communications are not always verbal; they are often experienced as sensations, images, or an inner knowing. This deep connection not only facilitates healing, but also strengthens the spiritual bond between the practitioner and the animal.

Integration is a crucial part of this process. After a healing session, it is important to give the animal time to rest and process the energies worked on. The Arcturians teach that animal healing does not always show immediate results, but the positive effects continue to integrate into their energy field over time.

The impact of this practice goes beyond the individual well-being of the animal. By working with the energies of these beings, the practitioner also contributes to the balance and harmony of the collective energy field. Animals, as natural guardians of the Earth, act as catalysts for high energies, and their healing benefits the entire ecosystem.

The Arcturians remind us that working with animals is an act of loving service, a reminder of the sacred connection between all life forms. Through animal healing, the practitioner not only promotes their well-being, but also participates in the creation of a more harmonious world, in alignment with higher frequencies.

This work is an expression of compassion and respect, an opportunity to deepen the relationship between humans and animals while contributing to universal energetic balance. Animal healing is not just a technique; it is a bridge to a deeper understanding of the interconnection of all life in the cosmos.

Chapter 22
Energy Protection and Release

Energy protection is an essential practice within the Arcturian holistic healing system, designed to preserve the integrity of the vibrational field against external influences that can disrupt its natural balance. The Arcturians teach that the environment, interactions with other people, and even certain thoughts and emotions can generate dense energies that affect physical, emotional, and spiritual well-being. Energy protection not only defends the practitioner's energy field but also strengthens their connection to higher frequencies.

The human energy field is dynamic and constantly interacts with the environment. However, when this field is exposed to discordant energies, cracks or blockages can form that diminish its vibration. Energy protection does not imply isolation, but rather establishing conscious vibrational boundaries that allow balanced interaction with the surroundings without compromising inner harmony.

The first step in energy protection is cleansing the vibrational field. This can be achieved through techniques such as visualization, conscious breathing, or the use of tools like crystals and herbs. For example, a practitioner can imagine a waterfall of golden light flowing from the top of the head to the feet, clearing any density or discordant energy. This act prepares the energy field to receive the necessary protection.

Visualizing energy shields is a central technique in this practice. During meditation, the practitioner can imagine themselves surrounded by a sphere of white or golden light that acts as a protective barrier. This shield allows the entry of high energies while blocking dense or negative influences. The Arcturians recommend reinforcing this visualization daily, especially before entering challenging environments.

The use of Arcturian symbols amplifies energy protection. Symbols such as the Star Tetrahedron or the Flower of Life can be visualized floating around the energy field, stabilizing it and creating a vibrational shield. These patterns not only protect but also harmonize and strengthen the practitioner's energy.

Crystals are valuable tools in energy protection. Stones such as black tourmaline, obsidian, and labradorite have properties that repel dense energies and seal the energy field. Placing one of these crystals in your pocket, wearing it as a pendant, or having it in the workplace reinforces the practitioner's protective barrier.

Sound is another effective technique for energy protection. Ringing a Tibetan bowl, using bells, or chanting mantras generates vibrations that cleanse and reinforce the energy field. For example, the mantra "OM" creates a resonance that balances and protects the practitioner's energy, creating a safe and vibrant space.

Conscious intention is an essential component of any energy protection practice. Before starting the day or facing energetically challenging situations, the practitioner can set a clear intention, such as "I am protected by divine light and my energy remains in balance." This act of intention not only directs the practitioner's energy but also strengthens their connection to higher frequencies.

Contact with nature is another way to protect and strengthen the energy field. Walking barefoot on the grass, hugging a tree, or meditating outdoors helps release discordant energies and reconnect with the natural flow of the Earth. The Arcturians teach that the Earth acts as a vibrational stabilizer, absorbing densities and recharging the practitioner's energy field.

Energy protection also includes conscious management of emotions and thoughts. Patterns of fear, anger, or anxiety generate cracks in the energy field, making it more vulnerable to external influences. Cultivating high vibrational emotions, such as gratitude, compassion, and love, strengthens the energy field and protects it from densities.

In interactions with other people, setting energetic boundaries is crucial. This can be achieved by visualizing a bubble of light around one's own energy field before intense encounters or internally remembering that each being is responsible for their own energy. This approach allows the practitioner to maintain their balance without absorbing the energies of others.

Integrating these practices into daily life ensures constant energy protection. The Arcturians remind us that consistency in these techniques strengthens the practitioner's energy field, making it more resilient and less susceptible to external influences. Even a few minutes a day dedicated to energy protection can have a significant impact on overall well-being.

Energy protection not only benefits the practitioner but also raises the vibration of their surroundings. A strong and balanced energy field acts as a beacon of light that radiates harmony to those around it, contributing to collective balance. This work is a reminder that energetic self-care is an act of service not only to oneself but also to the world.

The Arcturians teach that energy protection is not an act of separation, but a practice of empowerment. By keeping their vibrational field clean and protected, the practitioner becomes a clearer channel for higher frequencies, bringing light, balance, and healing to all levels of their life and those around them.

The release of energy blockages is an essential practice in the Arcturian holistic healing system, designed to restore the natural flow of energy in the body and the vibrational field. Blockages, which can manifest as physical tension, repressed emotions, or repetitive mental patterns, are accumulations of dense energy that disrupt the harmony of the system. By releasing them, the practitioner not only regains their balance but also accesses higher levels of well-being and consciousness.

The Arcturians teach that energy blockages are the result of unprocessed experiences, limiting beliefs, or external influences that have taken root in the system. Although these blocks may seem like obstacles, they are also opportunities for growth and transformation. The conscious release of these densities allows the practitioner to recover their natural energy flow and align with their higher purpose.

The first step in releasing blockages is identification. This requires conscious self-observation in which the practitioner reflects on areas of their life where they experience resistance, discomfort, or repetition of patterns. On a physical level, blockages can manifest as chronic pain or localized tension. Emotionally, they can present as anxiety, sadness, or persistent anger. Mentally, blockages often show up as recurring negative thoughts or self-imposed limitations.

Once a blockage is identified, the practitioner can use conscious breathing to begin dissolving it. During meditation, they can focus on the affected area, inhaling deeply and visualizing bringing light and energy to the blockage. Upon exhaling, they can imagine releasing the density, allowing the energy flow to be restored. This breathing cycle not only relaxes the system but also acts as a catalyst for vibrational transformation.

Guided visualization is a powerful technique in this process. The practitioner can imagine the blockage as a dark shape or a rigid structure in their energy field. While working with Arcturian energy, they can visualize this shape beginning to dissolve, transforming into vibrant light that flows freely through their system.

This technique not only releases the blockage but also restores harmony to the affected area.

Sound is another effective tool for releasing blockages. Using Tibetan bowls, bells, or mantras generates vibrations that penetrate deep into the energy field, disintegrating densities and allowing energy to flow again. During a session, the practitioner can ring a bell near the affected area, allowing the sound waves to interact with the blockage and release it.

Crystals are also valuable allies in this practice. Stones such as amethyst, obsidian, and citrine have properties that help transmute dense energies and restore energy balance. Placing a crystal on the area of the blockage or holding it during meditation amplifies the energy flow, facilitating release.

Laying on of hands is a central technique in Arcturian healing that can be used to release blockages. During a session, the practitioner can place their hands near the affected area, channeling Arcturian energy to the blockage. Visualizing a beam of golden light flowing from their hands to the area helps dissolve the density and restore balance.

Connecting with Arcturian frequencies significantly amplifies this work. During meditation, the practitioner can invoke these higher energies, visualizing a flow of vibrant light that penetrates the blockage and releases it. This light not only dissolves the density but also fills the released space with high frequencies, ensuring complete healing.

Conscious physical movement is another way to release energy blockages. Practices such as yoga, tai chi chuan, or even intuitive dance help to unblock areas where energy is stagnant, allowing it to flow freely again. Gentle movements combined with deep breathing amplify this effect, promoting release and harmonization.

Forgiveness is a transformative technique in releasing emotional blockages. Many densities are associated with emotional wounds or unresolved resentments. During meditation, the practitioner can visualize sending light and compassion to these experiences, releasing the associated emotional charge and restoring inner peace.

Integration is a crucial part of the release process. After working with a blockage, the practitioner should take time to rest, reflect, and allow the new energies to settle. The Arcturians teach that this integration time not only ensures that the release is complete but also strengthens the practitioner's energy field.

Releasing blockages not only transforms the practitioner but also raises their vibration, positively impacting their surroundings. By releasing densities, the practitioner radiates more harmonious energies, contributing to collective balance and planetary well-being.

The Arcturians remind us that releasing blockages is a continuous journey, an opportunity to grow, heal, and connect with our highest essence. By approaching these densities with compassion and openness, the practitioner not only restores their balance but also aligns with the higher frequencies that guide their path to wholeness and spiritual expansion.

Chapter 23
Healing Relationships and Light

Healing relationships is a transformative practice in the Arcturian holistic healing system, focused on harmonizing the energies shared between individuals, dissolving conflicts, and strengthening bonds from a perspective of love and understanding. The Arcturians teach that relationships, whether family, romantic, friendship, or professional, are a reflection of our internal energy field and a powerful tool for growth and spiritual evolution.

Each relationship has a unique energy, a vibrational flow that is generated and evolves as people interact. However, this flow can be altered by unresolved emotions, dysfunctional communication patterns, or external energies that affect the connection. Relationship healing does not seek to force changes in the people involved, but rather to transform the shared energies, promoting balance and alignment with the highest frequencies.

The first step in relationship healing is self-analysis. Before attempting to change the dynamics of a relationship, the practitioner should observe their own thoughts, emotions, and behavior patterns that may be contributing to conflicts or imbalances. This act of introspection not only generates clarity but also opens a space of responsibility and empowerment.

Meditation is a key tool for this process. During a meditative practice, the practitioner can visualize the energetic bond between themselves and the other person as a bond of light. If they perceive tensions or blockages in this bond, they can imagine a golden or pink light flowing towards it, clearing the densities and restoring harmony. This symbolic act reinforces the intention to heal and elevate the relationship.

Energy communication is another essential aspect of this practice. Through visualization, the practitioner can send vibrational messages of love, forgiveness, or gratitude to the other person. This not only affects the shared energy field, but also facilitates subtle changes in the dynamics of the relationship. The Arcturians emphasize that this communication must be carried out from a place of respect and compassion, without trying to manipulate or impose energies.

Forgiveness is a transformative component in relationship healing. Many tensions arise from past hurts or unresolved emotions. During a session, the practitioner can visualize sending light and compassion to the experiences shared with the other person, releasing resentments and allowing energies to flow freely again. This act not only heals the bond, but also frees the practitioner from emotional burdens.

Arcturian symbols are powerful tools for harmonizing relationships. During a practice, the practitioner can visualize a sacred symbol, such as the Flower of Life, rotating between themselves and the other person, balancing and strengthening the shared energy flow. These symbols act as vibrational matrices that elevate the connection and dissolve discordant energies.

Sound is another effective technique in relationship healing. Playing a Tibetan singing bowl or chanting mantras while visualizing the relationship can generate frequencies that cleanse and harmonize the bond. For example, chanting the mantra "OM" while focusing on the shared energetic bond can help dissolve tensions and restore balance.

Crystals can also be used to support relationship healing. Stones such as rose quartz, which resonates with unconditional love, or amethyst, which promotes clarity and peace, can be placed on an altar dedicated to the relationship or held during meditation. These crystals amplify the practitioner's intention and facilitate the transformation of the energetic bond.

Working with Arcturian frequencies amplifies the impact of this practice. During a session, the practitioner can invoke these higher energies, visualizing a ray of golden light flowing into the shared energetic bond. This light not only dissolves blockages and tensions, but also raises the vibration of the relationship, aligning it with the frequencies of love and understanding.

Introspective writing is a useful tool for exploring and healing relationship dynamics. The practitioner can reflect on questions such as "What lessons am I learning from this relationship?" or "What patterns do I want to transform in our connection?". Writing these reflections not only brings clarity, but also opens a space for introspection and healing.

Integration is an essential part of the relationship healing process. After working with the shared energies, it is important to observe how the bond and interactions feel. The Arcturians teach that energetic changes are often reflected in the physical world, but these may take time to fully manifest. Patience and consistency in practices ensure lasting transformation.

Relationship healing not only transforms personal connections, but also has a broader impact on the collective energy field. As the practitioner elevates their bonds, they radiate these frequencies to their surroundings, contributing to universal harmony and balance. This work is a reminder that each relationship is an opportunity to grow, learn, and expand unconditional love.

The Arcturians remind us that relationship healing is a path of self-discovery and connection, an invitation to transform our interactions into portals of spiritual growth and deep love. By approaching this work with intention, compassion, and openness, the practitioner not only restores harmony in their bonds, but also aligns with the higher frequencies that guide their evolution and spiritual expansion.

The transmission of light is a central practice in the Arcturian holistic healing system, designed to channel and share high frequencies with others, providing healing, clarity, and protection. The Arcturians teach that each human being has the ability to be a conscious channel of divine energy, transmitting light from the higher dimensions to the physical and spiritual planes. This practice not only helps the receiver to heal and raise their vibration, but also strengthens the practitioner, by integrating them with the higher frequencies and converting them into a conductor of peace and transformation.

The first step in the transmission of light is the conscious connection with the higher energies. Before carrying out any transmission work, the practitioner must align with their higher self, open their heart and mind, and establish a clear intention. This intention can be as simple as "I transmit light to heal and raise the energies of those who receive it" or "May the Arcturian light flow freely through me to restore harmony."

Conscious breathing plays a fundamental role in this practice. The practitioner should breathe deeply, inhaling the light from higher dimensions and visualizing how this light flows to their heart. Upon exhaling, the light radiates to the receiver, filling their energy field with healing frequencies. This rhythmic flow of breath reinforces the energy channel, ensuring that the transmission of light is fluid and harmonious.

The use of visualization is essential to amplify the transmission of light. During practice, the practitioner can imagine that their body is filled with a bright light, golden or white, representing divine energy. By extending their hands or directing their intention to the receiver, this light flows from their heart, enveloping the receiver in a healing energy field. The Arcturians teach that this light not only cleanses the receiver's energy field, but also aligns their physical, emotional, and spiritual bodies with the highest frequencies.

Arcturian symbols are powerful tools to amplify the transmission of light. During the session, the practitioner can visualize a sacred symbol floating above the receiver, transmitting healing energy through its geometric patterns. The use of symbols such as the Merkaba or the Star Tetrahedron can significantly enhance the frequency of the transmitted light, directing it precisely to the areas of the body or energy field that need healing.

Sound is also an important complement in the transmission of light. By chanting mantras, such as "OM" or channeled Arcturian sounds, the practitioner emits vibrations that reinforce the flow of light, further raising the receiver's frequencies. Sound resonates deeply in the subtle bodies, amplifying energy and helping to dissolve blockages and tensions. Instruments such as Tibetan singing bowls or bells are also effective, creating vibrations that allow light to flow more easily.

Working with crystals is another essential component of light transmission. Crystals such as clear quartz, selenite, or labradorite have properties that amplify healing energies. Placing a crystal in the practitioner's hands or near the receiver can intensify the transmitted energy, helping to direct light to specific areas that require attention. Crystals also act as amplifiers of Arcturian frequencies, ensuring that light flows with the greatest purity and power.

The transmission of light can be applied both in physical presence and at a distance. The Arcturians teach that energy work is not limited by physical barriers, and that energy can be effectively sent to anyone, anywhere in the world, through spiritual connection. For distance healing, the practitioner can visualize a bond of light connecting their energy field with that of the receiver. By imagining that light flows through this bond, energy reaches the receiver and provides them with healing, clarity, and protection, regardless of distance.

Energy protection is a crucial part of light transmission. Before sending energy to another being, the practitioner must ensure that their own energy field is protected and balanced. This can be achieved by visualizing a shield of light around the body, or by using protective crystals. Protection ensures that energy flows in a pure and interference-free manner, and that the practitioner's field remains in balance while acting as a channel of light.

The transmission of light is also an act of service. The Arcturians remind us that by sharing this energy with others, the practitioner not only helps to heal the receiver, but also connects with the universal network of light. By acting as channels of this divine energy, practitioners align more deeply with their spiritual purpose and contribute to collective well-being. The energy that is transmitted not only cleanses and heals, but also raises the vibration of the entire planet, creating a network of light that connects all beings.

Integration is essential when finishing a light transmission session. The practitioner should take time to rest, reflect, and allow the energies worked to settle.

This also applies to the receiver, who may experience a sense of peace and clarity after the transmission. Integrating these frequencies is essential for healing to become effective and to be maintained over time.

The transmission of light is a practice of universal love and compassion. The Arcturians teach that we all have the potential to be channels of this light and that, by doing so, we not only heal others, but also heal ourselves. By connecting with the higher energies and transmitting them, we restore balance in our own being and in the world around us, creating a continuous cycle of light and healing.

Chapter 24
Harmony with the Earth and Regeneration

Harmony with the Earth is an essential practice in the Arcturian holistic healing system, which recognizes the profound connection between human beings and the planet as a living, vibrant entity. The Arcturians teach that the Earth is not only our physical home, but also an energy field that nourishes and sustains all beings. Working in alignment with its rhythms and frequencies allows us to restore inner and outer balance, promoting personal and collective healing.

Connection with the Earth begins with understanding its energy as an expression of the universal flow. The Arcturians describe the Earth as a conscious being, a core of living energy that continuously responds and adapts to human and cosmic interactions. Establishing a harmonious relationship with this energy field not only benefits the practitioner, but also contributes to the overall well-being of the planet.

The first step in working with Earth's energy is the practice of grounding. This process allows the practitioner to balance their energy, stabilizing their system while strengthening their bond with the planet. During meditation, one can imagine roots of light extending from the feet to the Earth's core, absorbing its vibrant energy and returning any accumulated density. This bidirectional flow ensures a constant and harmonious exchange of energy.

Natural cycles, such as solstices, equinoxes, and lunar phases, are especially powerful times to align with Earth's frequencies. During these events, the practitioner can perform rituals or meditations that resonate with the energy of the moment. For example, on an equinox, one can focus on balancing their inner energies, reflecting the balance between light and darkness in nature.

The use of crystals is a powerful tool for working in harmony with the Earth. Stones such as black tourmaline, smoky quartz, and red jasper resonate with the frequencies of the Earth's core, acting as anchors that stabilize the practitioner's energy field. Placing these crystals on an altar, carrying them with you, or holding them during meditation amplifies the connection to the planet.

Direct contact with nature is fundamental to integrating this practice. Walking barefoot on the grass, meditating under a tree, or submerging in a natural body of water not only cleanses and balances the energy field, but also strengthens the connection with the living essence of the Earth. The Arcturians teach that these simple acts are gateways to a deeper relationship with the planet.

Sound is an effective vibrational tool for working with Earth's energies. Playing drums, using Tibetan bowls, or chanting specific mantras generates frequencies that resonate with the Earth's core. During a practice, the practitioner can visualize these vibrations extending to the Earth, connecting their energy field with the planet's flow.

Visualization is another powerful technique in this practice. During meditation, the practitioner can imagine themselves surrounded by a mantle of green or brown light, representing the Earth's energy. They can visualize this light flowing into their body, filling them with vitality, while they return love and gratitude to the planet. This exchange strengthens the relationship between the practitioner and the Earth, creating a deep energetic bond.

The practice of gratitude is central to harmony with the Earth. Expressing gratitude for the resources, beauty, and sustenance that the planet offers not only raises the vibration of the practitioner, but also contributes to the energetic healing of the Earth. During a session, the practitioner can dedicate a few moments to consciously give thanks for everything they receive from the natural environment.

Collective healing of the Earth is also an essential component of this practice. The Arcturians teach that humans have the power to send light and healing energy to the planet, contributing to its balance and regeneration. During meditation, the practitioner can visualize sending a beam of golden light from their heart to the planet, filling it with high frequencies that support its healing.

Integrating Arcturian frequencies amplifies the connection with the Earth. These higher energies act as a bridge between the practitioner and the planet's vibrational field, allowing for a deeper and more harmonious interaction. Invoking these frequencies during meditation or ritual practice intensifies healing and strengthens the spiritual connection with the Earth.

The Arcturians remind us that living in harmony with the Earth is not only a spiritual practice, but also an act of collective responsibility. By aligning with the planet's rhythms, the practitioner not only transforms their own energy, but also contributes to the balance and evolution of the entire ecosystem.

Harmony with the Earth is an invitation to remember our innate connection with the planet and act as conscious guardians of its energy. Through this practice, the practitioner not only restores their inner balance, but also becomes a channel of light and healing for the world around them, radiating frequencies of love and care to all life forms.

Regeneration techniques in the Arcturian holistic healing system are designed to activate the natural processes of restoration and renewal in the physical, emotional, and energetic body. These practices work in alignment with Arcturian frequencies, allowing the practitioner to stimulate the body's innate ability to heal, regenerate tissues, and restore balance at deep levels.

The Arcturians teach that regeneration is not just a biological process, but also an energetic flow that can be consciously activated. By working with these frequencies, the practitioner can access vibrational patterns that support cellular repair, emotional balance, and energy harmonization.

The first step in regeneration techniques is to connect with the body's life force. This involves a conscious focus on the areas that require regeneration, whether it is a physical wound, an unresolved emotion, or an imbalance in the energy field. The practitioner must establish a clear intention, such as "I activate my innate ability to heal and regenerate this area," to direct the energy effectively.

Conscious breathing is a fundamental tool in this process. During meditation, the practitioner can inhale deeply, visualizing Arcturian light flowing into the area that needs regeneration. As they exhale, they can imagine releasing any blockage or stagnant energy, allowing the regenerative flow to strengthen. This breathing cycle not only relaxes the body, but also activates the frequencies necessary for restoration.

The use of light and color is a powerful technique in regeneration. During a session, the practitioner can visualize a beam of golden, green, or blue light flowing into the area that needs healing. For example, green, associated with the energy of healing and balance, can be used to stimulate cellular repair, while blue can be used to soothe inflammation or tension.

Sacred geometry amplifies the impact of these practices. The practitioner can visualize patterns such as the Flower of Life or Metatron's Cube over the area that needs regeneration, allowing the frequencies of these symbols to activate and harmonize the tissues and energies involved. These patterns act as perfect matrices, guiding the energy flow to an optimal state of balance and renewal.

Crystals are valuable allies in regeneration techniques. Stones like clear quartz, green aventurine, and selenite have specific properties that support restoration and healing. Placing a crystal on the affected area or holding it during meditation amplifies the regenerative energy and reinforces the flow of Arcturian frequencies.

Sound is another effective vibrational tool. Using Tibetan bowls, tuning forks, or mantras generates frequencies that resonate deeply in the physical and energetic body, stimulating regeneration. For example, the mantra "RA MA DA SA", traditionally used for healing, can be chanted while focusing on the affected area, allowing the vibrations to activate restorative processes.

Conscious physical contact, such as the laying on of hands, is also an essential technique. During a session, the practitioner can place their hands on the affected area, channeling Arcturian energy into it. Visualizing a flow of golden or emerald light flowing from their hands into the area not only stimulates regeneration, but also strengthens the bond between the physical body and the energy field.

Working with Arcturian frequencies is at the core of these techniques. During a practice, the practitioner can invoke these higher energies, visualizing a field of vibrant light that envelops their entire body or focuses on specific areas. These frequencies not only stimulate regeneration at the cellular level, but also balance the energy field, ensuring holistic restoration.

Emotional regeneration is a key component of these practices. Many physical ailments are linked to unprocessed emotions that have become stored in the body. During a session, the practitioner can explore the emotions associated with the affected area, using techniques such as forgiveness or emotional release to support regeneration.

Integration is a crucial part of the regenerative process. After a session, the practitioner should take time to rest, hydrate, and allow the energies worked with to settle. Regeneration does not always occur immediately, but the activated frequencies continue to work in the body and energy field for days or weeks.

The Arcturians teach that regeneration techniques not only transform the individual, but also contribute to collective well-being. By restoring their own balance, the practitioner raises their vibration and becomes a channel of harmonious energies for their surroundings. This work is a reminder that personal regeneration and planetary healing are intrinsically connected.

The practice of regeneration techniques is an invitation to rediscover and activate the body's innate potential to heal and renew itself. Through these techniques, the practitioner not only transforms their personal experience, but also aligns with higher frequencies, remembering their ability to co-create well-being, balance, and wholeness at all levels of existence.

Chapter 25
Child and Group Healing

Working with children within the Arcturian holistic healing system is a practice that requires sensitivity, intuition, and a loving approach. Children have a purer and more open energetic field than adults, which allows them to respond quickly to high frequencies. However, they are also more sensitive to external influences, which makes them susceptible to energetic imbalances that can manifest in their behavior, emotions, or physical health.

The Arcturians teach that working with children is a sacred opportunity to support their well-being and foster their connection to higher energies from an early age. This work not only benefits the child, but also strengthens the energetic bond between the practitioner, the child, and their environment, promoting family and collective harmony.

The first step in working with children is to create a safe and welcoming space where they can feel relaxed and open to the experience. This space should be peaceful, with an atmosphere that invites calm and curiosity. Elements such as soft lighting, relaxing music, and warm colors can help create a harmonious environment.

The initial connection with the child should be intuitive and based on trust. Before starting any energy practice, the practitioner can take a few moments to observe and understand the child's energy, respecting their level of comfort and openness. Children are receptive to intentions and emotions, so it is essential that the practitioner focuses on radiating calm, love, and security.

Healing techniques for children should be adapted to their needs and level of understanding. Instead of detailed explanations, the practitioner can use stories, images, or games that allow them to connect with energies in a natural way. For example, the child can be invited to imagine a bright, warm light surrounding them, like a protective hug from the universe.

Visualization is a powerful tool in working with children. The practitioner can guide them to imagine colors and shapes that convey tranquility and well-being. For example, they can be asked to visualize a rainbow flowing through their body, cleansing and balancing their energy. These simple and visually appealing images are easy to understand and deeply effective.

Mindful breathing can be taught as a game for children. They can be asked to imagine that they are inhaling stars or flowers and exhaling clouds or bubbles. This approach not only introduces the concept of mindful breathing, but also helps them release tension and balance their energy in a playful way.

Gentle physical contact is an especially effective technique with children. Placing your hands on their head, back, or hands while channeling Arcturian frequencies can help calm their system and restore balance. During this process, the practitioner can visualize a golden or emerald light flowing from their hands to the child's body, filling them with calm and well-being.

The use of tools such as crystals is also very well received by children, as they tend to be attracted to their beauty and energy. Crystals such as rose quartz, amethyst, or green aventurine are ideal for working with children due to their gentle and protective properties. You can give a crystal for them to hold or place it nearby while conducting the session.

Sound is another vibrational tool that resonates deeply with children. Using instruments such as bells, small drums, or Tibetan bowls creates a magical environment that children find fascinating. These sounds not only balance their energy, but also stimulate their curiosity and creativity.

Play is a natural way to work with children's energies. The Arcturians suggest that imaginative games, such as creating "shields of light" or "magical energy portals", can be an effective way to introduce concepts of protection and balance. Through play, children not only understand the practices, but also actively participate in their own healing.

It is important that sessions are short and dynamic, adapting to the child's attention span. Children tend to respond quickly to energies, so it is not necessary to spend a long time to achieve significant effects. At the end, the practitioner can guide them to express how they feel, encouraging self-exploration and self-knowledge.

Emotional support is also essential in working with children. Often, unbalanced energies are associated with unexpressed emotions or changes in their environment. Listening carefully and validating their feelings strengthens their confidence and provides them with a safe space to process their experiences.

The impact of working with children transcends the moment of the session. The Arcturians teach that children who feel balanced and connected to their inner energy tend to radiate this harmony to their surroundings. This creates an expansive healing effect that benefits their families, schools, and communities.

Working with children is an opportunity to sow the seeds of well-being and spiritual connection from an early age. The Arcturians remind us that children are bearers of light and innate wisdom, and that by supporting them in their energetic balance and development, we not only contribute to their well-being, but also to the creation of a more harmonious and elevated future for all.

The development of healing groups within the context of the Arcturian holistic healing system is a practice that combines individual and collective intentions to amplify the impact of healing energies. The Arcturians teach that groups act as energetic nodes that, when united, create a larger vibrational field capable of healing, transforming, and uplifting both the participants and the environment that surrounds them. This practice not only strengthens the connection between members, but also contributes to collective balance and planetary well-being.

The formation of a healing group begins with a clear intention shared by all participants. The purpose can range from the individual healing of its members to the transmission of healing energies to specific communities or places. Defining this intention together aligns the group's energies and establishes a solid foundation for spiritual work.

The first practical step is to create a sacred space where the group can gather. This space should be peaceful, harmonious, and conducive to meditation and energetic connection. Elements such as candles, crystals, soft music, and sacred symbols can be strategically placed to raise the vibration of the place and create an environment that inspires calm and concentration.

The energetic preparation of the participants is fundamental to the success of the group. Before starting any practice, it is recommended to perform grounding exercises, energy cleansing, and individual alignment. This ensures that each member contributes with a balanced energy field and is open to receiving and transmitting Arcturian frequencies.

Group meditation is one of the most powerful practices in this context. During the session, participants can visualize a golden sphere of light surrounding them, connecting their energies and creating a unified vibrational field. This sphere acts as a channel that amplifies shared intentions and facilitates the flow of healing energies both within and outside the group.

Channeling Arcturian frequencies is a central element in healing groups. One or more participants can act as conscious channels, receiving and transmitting these energies to the rest of the group. Visualizing a ray of golden light descending from the higher dimensions to the center of the group circle is an effective technique to activate and distribute these frequencies.

The use of sacred geometry amplifies the effectiveness of group practices. Patterns such as the Flower of Life or the Star Tetrahedron can be visualized floating in the center of the group, radiating balancing energy to all members. These symbols can also be drawn or physically placed in space, serving as focal points for Arcturian energies.

Sound is another transformative tool in healing groups. Using Tibetan bowls, drums, or bells creates vibrations that resonate with the group's energy field, harmonizing and raising its frequency. Mantras, such as "OM" or "RA MA DA SA", can be chanted together, synchronizing the energies of the participants and strengthening the collective connection.

Working with crystals is especially effective in groups. Placing a large crystal, such as a clear quartz or amethyst, in the center of the circle amplifies and distributes healing energies. Participants can also hold smaller crystals during sessions, establishing a direct connection with Arcturian frequencies.

The collective intention can be directed towards specific goals, such as sending light and healing to a person, community, or situation. During these practices, group members can visualize the intention as a ray of light flowing from the center of the circle to the target, carrying with it the healing and transformative energies generated by the group.

Group dynamics should include time to share experiences and reflections after practices. This space allows participants to express what they felt or perceived, strengthening the emotional and spiritual connection between members. The Arcturians teach that this interaction not only enriches the individual experience, but also deepens the energetic cohesion of the group.

Developing roles within the group can be helpful in organizing and optimizing practices. Some members may assume the role of facilitators, guiding meditations and energy practices, while others may focus on logistical aspects or preparing the sacred space. This collaborative approach strengthens the sense of shared purpose and ensures that each participant contributes their unique talents.

Regularity in meetings is essential to maintain the consistency and effectiveness of the group. Establishing a fixed schedule, such as weekly or monthly meetings, creates a rhythm that strengthens the energetic connection between members. The Arcturians teach that consistency in these practices not only deepens the impact of the energies worked with, but also raises the vibration of the environment and communities connected to the group.

Healing groups also have an impact beyond their immediate members. The Arcturians emphasize that collective work generates an expansive wave of light that contributes to the balance and healing of the planet. This multiplier effect transforms the group into a catalyst for positive change, radiating high frequencies to all dimensions of existence.

The development of healing groups is a manifestation of the interconnection between human beings and their ability to co-create harmony and well-being. Through these practices, participants not only transform their own energy, but also contribute to a greater purpose, aligning themselves with Arcturian frequencies to promote healing and balance in the world.

Chapter 26
Mastery and Advanced Practice

Advancements in the practice of the Arcturian holistic healing system represent a higher step on the path of personal and collective transformation.

The Arcturians teach that true mastery in healing lies not only in technical knowledge, but in the ability to adapt the learned tools to the unique needs of each situation. Advanced practice is, therefore, an intuitive dance between acquired skills and the spiritual guidance that the practitioner receives in each moment.

The first step in these advancements is to deepen the connection with Arcturian frequencies. Through more intense and prolonged meditations, the practitioner can refine their ability to perceive and channel these energies with greater clarity. Visualizing a vortex of golden light descending from higher dimensions, enveloping the body and the energy field, helps to open new levels of perception and sensitivity.

The combination of techniques is one of the pillars of advanced practice. For example, the practitioner can integrate sacred geometry with sound, using patterns such as the Flower of Life while chanting specific mantras. This synergy enhances the impact of both tools, allowing the practitioner to address more complex and profound energy blocks.

Personalization of techniques is also key. Instead of applying general methods, the practitioner must tune in to the unique energy of the person, place, or situation they are working with. This may involve adjusting the frequency of the visualized light, choosing specific crystals according to the detected needs, or adapting visualizations and meditations to address specific energetic aspects.

Multidimensional work is a central aspect of advancements in practice. The Arcturians teach that many energetic imbalances have roots in dimensions beyond the physical plane. During a session, the practitioner can visualize themselves entering an elevated vibrational space, where they work directly with timelines, Akashic memories, or ancestral energies that influence the present.

Collective healing is another area of expansion in advanced practice. When working with groups or communities, the practitioner must be able to direct energy simultaneously to multiple individuals, maintaining a clear and stable focus. Visualizing an interweaving of light connecting all participants allows the Arcturian frequencies to be distributed evenly, strengthening the impact of group healing.

The use of advanced symbols is a powerful technique at this stage. The Arcturians teach that each symbol has a specific vibrational pattern that can be activated through conscious intention. During a session, the practitioner can visualize a symbol floating above the area being worked on, rotating and expanding to direct energy with precision. Incorporating new symbols discovered through meditation and channeling enriches the practitioner's repertoire and allows them to address more specific challenges.

Mastery of energy flow is another essential component. At this stage, the practitioner must be able to perceive the movement of energy in real time, detecting areas of congestion or imbalance and adjusting their focus as needed. This requires a high level of sensitivity and a constant connection to the higher energies that guide the session.

The integration of emotions and mental patterns also plays an important role in advanced practice. Often, energy blocks are deeply linked to repressed emotions or limiting beliefs. During a session, the practitioner can invite the recipient to explore and release these emotions, using techniques such as visualizing transforming light or using positive affirmations that reprogram the energy field.

The use of intuition is essential at this level. The Arcturians teach that each healing session is unique and requires a personalized response that cannot always be planned in advance. Trusting inner impulses, visualized images, and sensations perceived during practice allows the practitioner to act as a clear channel for Arcturian frequencies.

Self-assessment and continuous development are also crucial at this stage. The Arcturians emphasize the importance of constant practice, daily meditation, and seeking new ways to expand knowledge and skill.

Reflecting on each session, identifying what worked and what can be improved, allows the practitioner to refine their approach and advance on their spiritual path.

Advanced practice not only transforms the practitioner, but also amplifies their impact on the world. The Arcturians teach that those who work with these higher frequencies not only heal and balance others, but also raise the vibration of the collective. Each healing session, each transmission of light, and each conscious interaction contribute to universal balance.

Advancements in practice are an invitation to take acquired skills to a new level of mastery, where intuition, sensitivity, and connection to Arcturian frequencies combine to address complex challenges with grace and precision. This path not only deepens the practitioner's connection to higher energies, but also aligns them with their purpose as a channel of light and healing in the world.

Becoming an Arcturian Master is the culmination of a journey of learning, practice, and transformation in the Arcturian holistic healing system. This state is not defined solely by technical mastery, but by the deep integration of Arcturian frequencies into all aspects of the practitioner's life. An Arcturian Master acts as a bridge between the higher dimensions and the earthly plane, serving as a guide, healer, and bearer of light for those seeking harmony and balance.

The Arcturians teach that mastery is a continuous process, a commitment to growth and expansion. It is not about reaching an end point, but about being in a constant state of receptivity and service. This path requires humility, discipline, and a deep respect for the higher energies that guide each step of the practitioner.

The first step towards mastery is complete alignment with Arcturian frequencies. This implies not only the ability to channel these energies during healing practices, but also to integrate them into daily life. An Arcturian Master lives in a state of constant connection with these frequencies, allowing them to guide their thoughts, words, and actions.

Conscious presence is an essential quality of an Arcturian Master. This ability allows the practitioner to be fully present in each moment, perceiving the subtle energies around them and responding with clarity and compassion. The daily practice of meditation and self-observation strengthens this capacity, creating a stable and luminous energy field that radiates balance towards others.

Teaching is one of the fundamental responsibilities of an Arcturian Master. Sharing the knowledge and techniques learned not only benefits those who receive them, but also strengthens the Master's connection to higher energies. A true master does not impose their wisdom, but inspires and guides, allowing each individual to discover their own path towards healing and enlightenment.

Service is another essential aspect of mastery. The Arcturians emphasize that an Arcturian Master acts for the benefit of the collective, using their skills and knowledge to uplift others. This may include individual healing, transmitting light to communities, or working with groups to harmonize collective energies. Service is not an obligation, but a natural expression of love and gratitude towards the energies that the Master channels.

Connection with the Arcturian Masters is a central part of this stage. These spiritual guides offer guidance, support, and wisdom to those who have reached advanced levels in their practice. During meditations, an Arcturian Master can visualize a circle of light where these guides meet, receiving their energy and messages to deepen their own understanding and expansion.

Mastery of advanced techniques is a distinctive characteristic of an Arcturian Master. This includes the ability to work with multidimensional energies, energy reprogramming, interdimensional healing, and activation of the light body. A Master not only uses these techniques with precision, but also adapts and expands them according to the needs of each situation.

Inner balance is fundamental to maintaining the state of mastery. The Arcturians teach that an Arcturian Master must be an example of harmony, demonstrating how higher energies can be integrated into everyday life. This includes conscious management of emotions, positive thinking, and the ability to maintain a high vibration even in challenging circumstances.

Energy protection is also crucial for an Arcturian Master. When working with high energies and assisting others in their healing processes, the Master must ensure that they keep their own energy field clean and balanced. This can be achieved through visualizations, protective crystals, Arcturian symbols, and regular energy cleansing practices.

The creation of communities of light is another important aspect of mastery. An Arcturian Master not only works individually, but also inspires and organizes groups to promote collective healing and upliftment. These communities act as focal points of light, radiating high frequencies towards their members and the surrounding environment.

The legacy of an Arcturian Master is not measured by their individual achievements, but by the impact they have on others. The Arcturians teach that a true Master leaves a mark of light and love in all their interactions, reminding those around them of their own connection to higher energies and their ability to transform.

Humility is the foundation of mastery. An Arcturian Master understands that they are not the source of the energies they channel, but an instrument at the service of the universe. This recognition allows Arcturian frequencies to flow freely through them, creating a clear and powerful channel for healing and transformation.

Becoming an Arcturian Master is an invitation to live in constant alignment with the highest frequencies, serving as a beacon of light for the world. This path not only transforms the practitioner, but also uplifts all those with whom they interact, creating a network of light that connects hearts, minds, and souls in a common purpose of love, healing, and unity.

Epilogue

As you reach the end of these pages, you are no longer the same. Something subtle, yet profoundly transformative, has changed within you. It may be difficult to identify exactly what, but if you listen carefully, you will feel that the melody that now vibrates in your essence is clearer, more tuned, more connected to the whole.

The journey you began when you opened this book does not end here. It is a starting point, an opening to dimensions that previously seemed unattainable. You have not only accessed knowledge, but also frequencies that continue to reverberate in your energy system. And this is just the beginning.

The Arcturians, with their wisdom and presence, do not offer definitive answers, but tools for you to find your own. They show the way, but it is you who decides to walk it. It is an invitation to co-creation, to active participation in the healing and expansion of your own reality.

Remember that true healing, true balance, lies in recognizing the interconnection of all that you are. Body, mind, and spirit are like a sacred triangle, and when one is in harmony, all the others align. Your life now reflects this harmony, and the energy you radiate has the power to transform not only your being, but also those around you.

As you close this book, know that it will never be completely closed. It remains alive within you, in every practice you decide to adopt, in every intention you set, in every moment you choose to vibrate at a higher frequency. This is your legacy: a continuous awakening, an eternal dance between you and the universe.

Go forth, with courage and an open heart. The cosmos is by your side. And within you is the key to everything.

www.ingramcontent.com/pod-product-compliance
Lightning Source LLC
LaVergne TN
LVHW040051080526
838202LV00045B/3578